THE MANBASICS GUIDE TO A KICK ASS BEARD

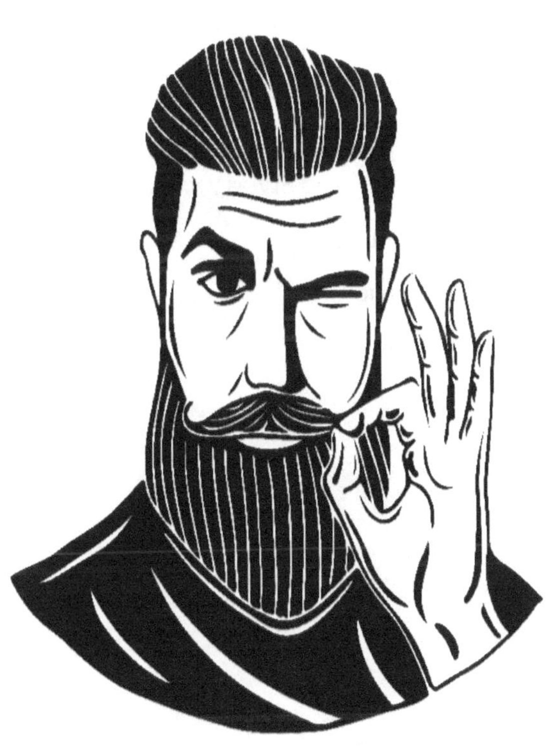

Table of Contents

Table of Contents

Introduction

"Your beard itches when you kiss me. Are you sure you want to keep it?"

Guys, after being married for twenty-plus years I can tell you that I have finally deciphered that seemingly foreign and nonsensical sentence.   Roughly translated she is saying:

"Your beard sucks. It looks like a rat crawled onto your face and died. Fix it or get rid of it. And take out the garbage while you're at it."

The thing is, she was totally right. Twelve years ago or so when she first said that, I had no idea what I was doing. It would likely be called "not shaving" more than "growing a beard." It appeared that all I was growing were seeds of discontentment with my sex life.

Naturally, I shaved the damn thing quick.

Fast forward to a few years ago. I gave it a go and THIS time I told her "I'm the man of the house and if I want a damn beard I'm gonna have a damn beard . . ."

OK, that sentence is a lot easier to type than it is to speak out loud, and it is obviously a total lie. To be honest with you, I looked over my shoulder as I typed that sentence to ensure she wasn't looking. Love you, honey!

No, what REALLY happened is she was going out of town for a week. Being that it was "Mo-vember," I thought it would be the perfect time to give it another go. After all, she had said, "fix it, or get rid of it." So why not try Door Number One?

I even planned ahead and got a couple days' head start by not shaving for a few days before she left. This time around I was going to do it right and do some homework on how to actually style and maintain a beard and moustache.

I had heard a rumor that the Internet could be used for something besides food porn, actual porn, and cat memes.

What I ended up finding was the beginning of the tome you hold in your hands right now. I'm not going to sell you some load of bullshit that I'm a master stylist, have won a beard competition, or hell . . . even that I have a great-looking beard.

I WILL tell you that when my wife came home, we had a four-day weekend romp that would have made Prince blush (or the Artist Formerly Known as…?).

Just kidding again. We'd been married for twenty years at this point.   might as well tell you she brought home a unicorn. But I can tell you that she did say, "Huh . . . you grew your beard again."

I responded that yes, I had in fact grown my beard so as to celebrate Mo-vember.   I further commented that I would probably shave it in December or by the first of the year.

Anyway, that was a couple years ago and here I still am with my beard so I must have done SOMETHING right. In fact, after a couple of months, I really WAS going to shave it. But my wife said, "Nah don't, I kinda like it now."

Guys, I rest my case here: "I kinda like it now."   To translate "wife speak" into "guy speak": "You are the man in my life. Take me now you hunk of masculine man flesh."

So like I said, I'm no technical expert on this stuff. I'm more like a beard curator. There's a lot of great information out there on beard-growing and maintaining best practices, but it IS all pretty spread out. This humble submission is my contribution to the beard community. I hope it meets with your approval.

Cheers, and happy growing!

Damon Henrichs

Spring, TX 10/7/19

Chapter One – A Brief History of Beards, Part One

And I do mean brief. To go into a detailed history here would literally start with Adam (Eve evidently didn't think Adam's beard was scratchy when THEY kissed), and could end with James Harden.

Seriously though, Adam almost certainly had a beard, right? Where the hell would he have gotten a razor? Or a knife? Using a sharp rock seems a little extreme . . .

It does beg the question though, how DID early man shave exactly? Or WHY even? After all, having a beard is clearly our natural state of being.

Frankly, the early history of the beard is less a history of the beard so much as it is a history of SHAVING. In the ancient world, shaving would have been expensive, time-consuming, and it would have taken someone of influence to decide it was a really cool thing to do. Someone cool enough that thousands of others would have said "F yeah, shave it, baby!"

To address each objection in turn, let's start with cost. As I mentioned, in the beginning there were rocks. And God looked at the rocks and said "Let there be shaving cream powerful enough that a sharp rock won't hurt like the dickens when someone tries to shave with one."

Unfortunately, that verse in Genesis was lost to history which means that Adam, and pretty much everyone up to the Bronze Age had to do without shaving of any real kind. Maybe they used said rock to trim up their hair, their beard, and even their pubes if they were confident in their ability with the rock, but actual shaving? Not so much.

Or DID they?

Believe it or not, sharp rocks quite possibly WERE used as primitive razors. Evidence that early man sharpened clam shells, shark teeth, and flint have been found dating as far back as 30,000 years! You can even find a video of a modern man shaving with obsidian to demonstrate this principal. It's likely that early man would have used various animal fats in place of shaving cream. How prevalent this would have been brings me to my second area of objection: time.

If you think it takes time to shave every day in the 21st century just imagine what an enormous pain in the ass it would have been to shave with obsidian glass and some whale blubber. Not to mention there was no such thing as a mirror, which makes it likely that in order to shave you actually had to have someone else shaving your face for you (or a tremendously helpful spouse volunteering to you that "you missed a spot").

While we can't know for sure, it seems likely that shaving was a luxury for the wealthy with a full load of "nothing better to do" on their hands.

In short, beards likely were styled in the classic "Hey I dunno, it just grew like this . . ." style and shaven faces probably were seen, but likely more common among the wealthy.

Romans and Bronze

It seems that the earliest truly "man-made" razors were made of bronze by the Egyptians. While I am speculating that shaving would have been for the wealthy in prehistoric times, it is almost certain this was the case in Egypt, because razors made of bronze have been found.

Bronze doesn't come from the ground like iron does. Bronze is a combination of copper and tin. I won't bore you with the specifics, but trust me . . . in ancient Egypt, this was expensive.

So once again you have the "have's" deciding to "have not" a beard, while the "have nots" totally are rocking beards like they were 4,500 years early for a ZZ Top audition.

Alexander The Great

All that changed with the arrival of Alexander the Great. Despite being totally great, there seems to be something he was not so great at, and that was growing facial hair. Or, if you believe the Oliver Stone movie, Alexander preferred the [ahem] "boyish" look.

Whatever the reason, there is little doubt that Alexander preferred his army clean-shaven. Alexander's Macedonians are said to have shaved because he believed a beard could be grabbed in battle, so it was a battle advantage to be clean-shaven.

He may have been onto something since he pretty much conquered the entire known world by the age of 30. Or it might have been the shoes. At any rate, it is clear the Macedonians shaved because Alexander wanted them to.

After Alexander, pretty much all bets were off when it came to shaving. The Romans followed suit in preferring to be clean-shaven, likely in some form of hero worship of Alexander. There's no real evidence for that, but there's also no real evidence of why Romans decided to shave in the first place. The fact that Rome decided to ALSO go and conquer the entire known world makes me believe I might be onto something with my shot in the dark speculation.

Snip Snip

The rest is pretty much history (OK, all the stuff before was history too, but who's keeping track). From as early on as Romans and Egyptians, it had been established that man could choose to have a beard, or choose NOT have a beard.

From there, of course, it was only a matter of time before man began exploring the full range of awesomeness that is the human beard. The biggest determinant here was the technology, which would allow such experimentation to take place. A beard meant no shaving, a primitive razor meant shaving ... but what about all the awesome-sauce in between?

THAT my friend, requires scissors.

Scissors have a history similar to that of razors, but less ancient. Evidence of some bronze scissors dates as far back as 3000 BC. As I mentioned before with the razor, bronze was a rich substance not for the everyday schmuck. And unlike the razor, scissors would have required quite a bit more expertise to craft. They were "spring scissors" whereby the two blades are held together by a curved piece of bronze that allows it to "spring" back open again.

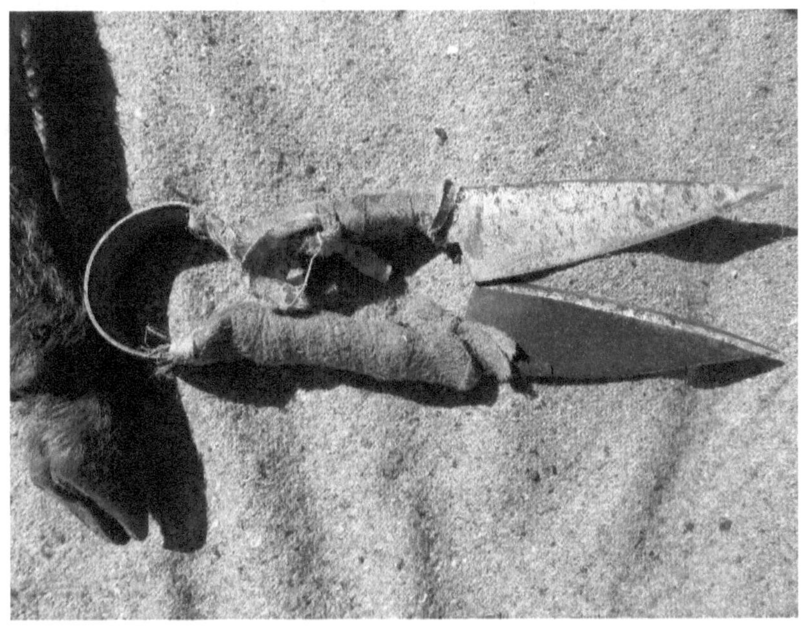

Figure 1 - Ancient bronze spring scissors from Egypt.

These spring scissors were the norm all the way until about the mid 18th century. This coincides almost to the decade with the invention of a razor for the masses. The first modern straight razor complete with decorated handles and hollow ground blades was constructed in Sheffield, England--the center of the cutlery industry, in the 18th and 19th centuries.

FINALLY, the common man had unfettered access to some serious beard maintenance! It's no wonder that the 18th and 19th centuries are when we start to see paintings and photographs of some of the more epic beard and moustache styles we have come to know and love today: the handlebar, the sideburn (more on that later!), the Balbo, The Circle Beard, The Imperial…the list goes on!

Chapter Two – A Brief History of Beards, Part Two

There's really not much more to say about the actual history of the beard without making it some sort of history book, and I doubt that's why you decided to read this.

That said, there is some more history to be told in simply calling out and paying homage to some of the greatest, famous (infamous in some cases), and most epic beards in history.

Leonardo Da Vinci – Da Vinci was the O.G, or more specifically…the O.R. M. – Original Renaissance Man. Here's a guy renowned for his ability in sculpting, painting, human anatomy, engineering, math, architecture, and a whole host of random inventions (yeah, in his "spare time" he invented The Helicopter). So OF COURSE he had an amazing beard. Da Vinci's famous beard grew all the way down to his mid-sternum and was reputed to be nearly as wide as his shoulders.

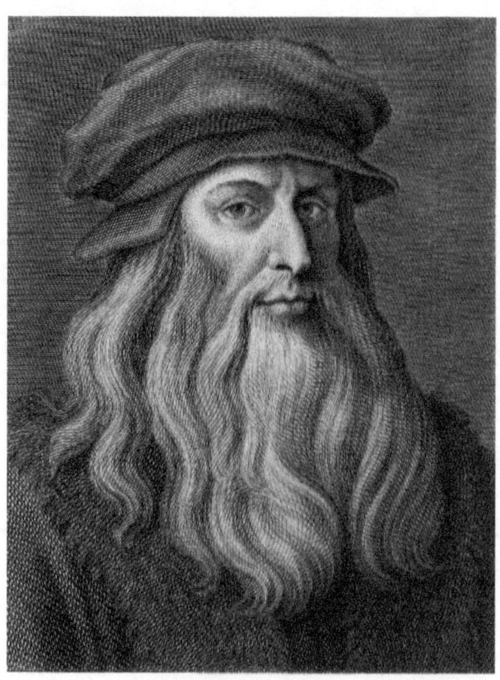

Figure 2 - Leonardo Da Vinci looking dapper as the Original Renaissance Man

Johannes Brahms – Classical composer Johannes Brahms was said to be the continuing legacy of Beethoven (his 1st Symphony is sometimes called "Beethoven's 10th Symphony). Brahms was known in his time to be a perfectionist with his work, and it certainly showed up in his glorious beard. It's almost as if a Persian Long Hair Feline curled up on his face and made residence there. Brahms wrote the famous "lullaby" melody, so next time you are having trouble sleeping try humming that melody and counting amazing beards until you drift off. You will either be happily out like a light or jumping out of bed to examine your own (likely inferior) beard in the mirror.

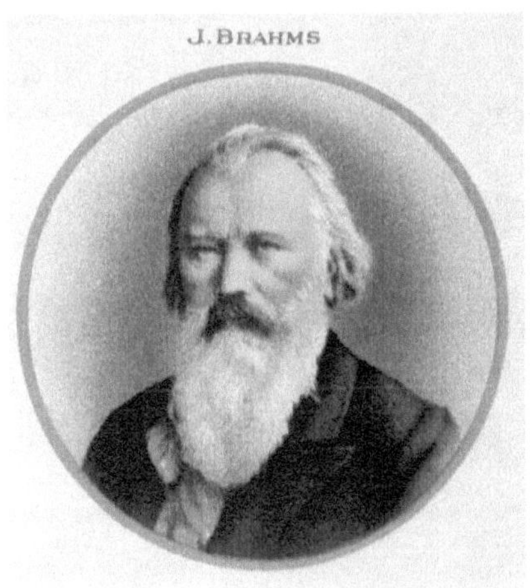

Figure 3 - Johannes Brahms - His beard was as epic as his music.

Karl Marx – All beards are equal, but some are more equal than others. Marx's beard was not only full and bushy, but sported a recognizable and decidedly darker moustache than the rest of his facial hair. Whatever you may think of his politics there is no denying that this was a beard for the ages, which he himself referred to as his "Prophet's Beard." There are 15 known photos of Karl Marx, and he sports an impressive crumb duster in all of them.

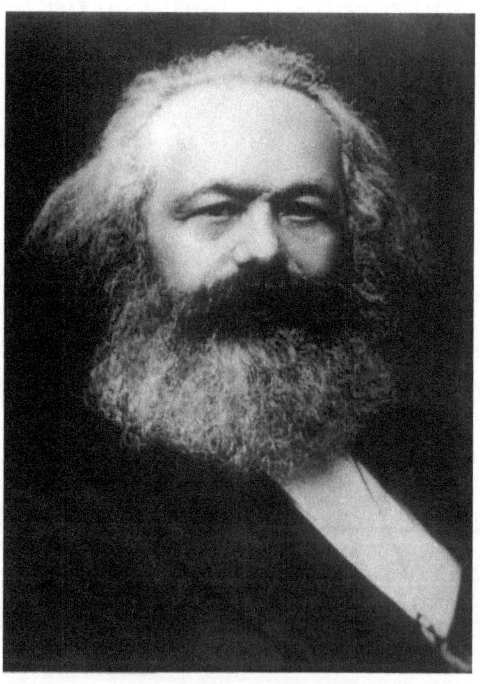

Figure 4 - Karl Marx. Would he have considered sharing part of his beard with other less fortunate bearded brothers?

Rasputin – Rasputin was a bearded mystic who rose from the ranks of peasant to trusted advisor to Czar Nicholas the 2nd, due in large part to his mastery of mysticism and faith healing. I like to think Rasputin simply walked in and said, "See this beard? I grew it through the power of mysticism" and then the Czar nodded sagely and said, "You're hired." Either that or it was his crazy eyes.

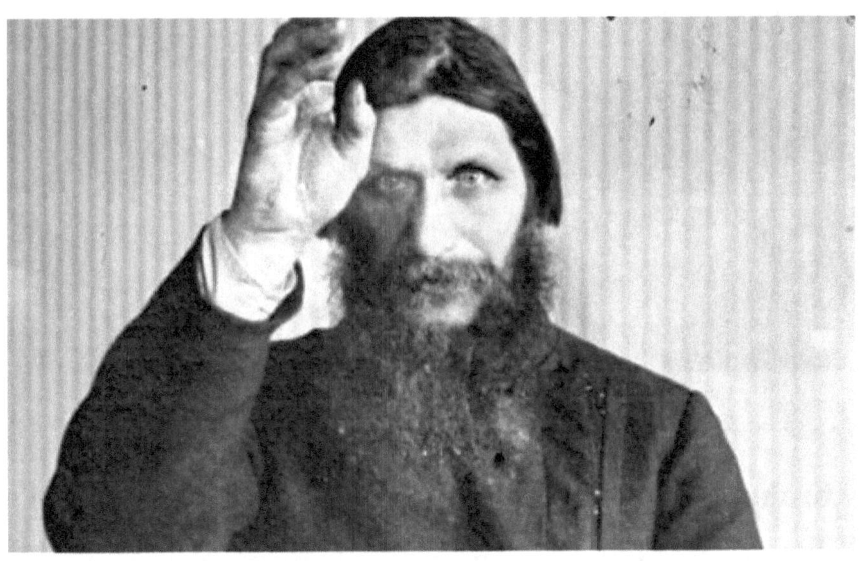

Figure 5 - Rasputin, holy crap those crazy eyes!

Wyatt Earp and Doc Holiday – OK, so sure these two gents are known more for moustaches and not beards…but they are freaking iconic and epic as well as a contrast in two styles, just like the two western gunslingers themselves. We won't rehash their entire story here, go watch "Tombstone" if you want that. We just couldn't let a list like this go without at least a solemn nod to their amazing lip foliage.

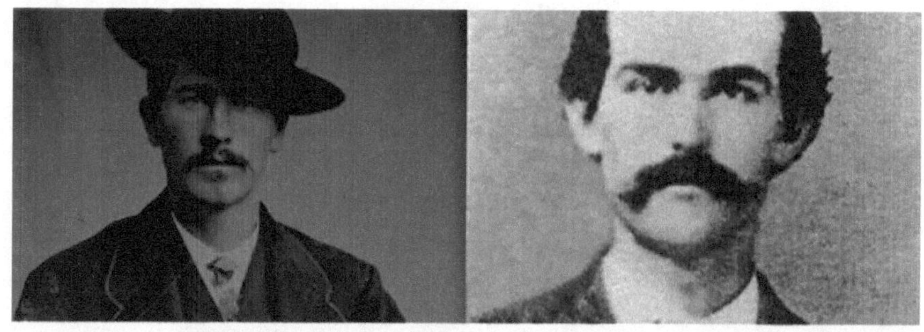

Figure 6 - Wyatt Earp and Doc Holiday.   He's your Huckleberry.

Abraham Lincoln – So we already talked about Lincoln and how he pretty much inspired every general in the Union AND Confederate army to sport epic chin guards. While certainly a respectable beard unto itself, the brilliance of Lincoln's beard lies more in its sheer recognizability. Check him out WITHOUT a beard. Hardly looks like the same person. Incidentally, Lincoln had lived most of his life WITHOUT a beard. Shortly before the 1860 election an eleven year-old girl wrote Lincoln, "let your whiskers grow… [as] you would look a great deal better for your face is so thin". THAT is a smart damn kid.

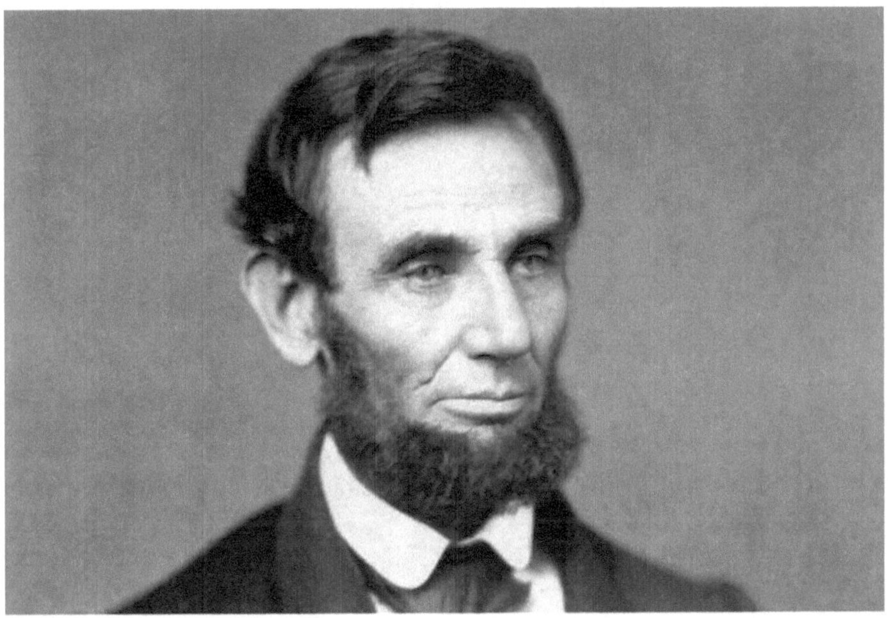

Figure 7 - Abraham Lincoln: Four Score and Seven Beards Ago . . .

Ambrose Burnside – You KNOW you have an important beard when an entire style of beard is named after you. Yes, the "sideburn" is a play on Ambrose Burnside's name. Civil War enthusiasts will say Burnside was not much of a general for the Union. Beard enthusiasts will say, "You shut your damn mouth!"

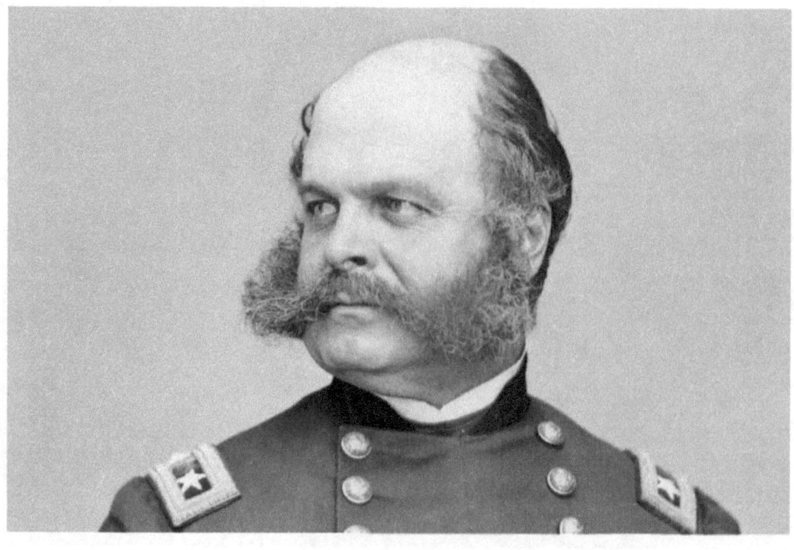

Figure 8 -Ambrose Burnside. You may be cool, but you will likely never be "Had a style of beard named after you" cool.

Salvadore Dali – Another non-beard entry, but how can you deny giving Salvadore some credit? A talented surrealist painter who clearly brought his style, art, and sense of humor to his moustache. He even co-wrote a book ABOUT his moustache called (wait for it) "Dali's Moustache." Evidently his book title writing was a little less inspired than his art, or his moustache.

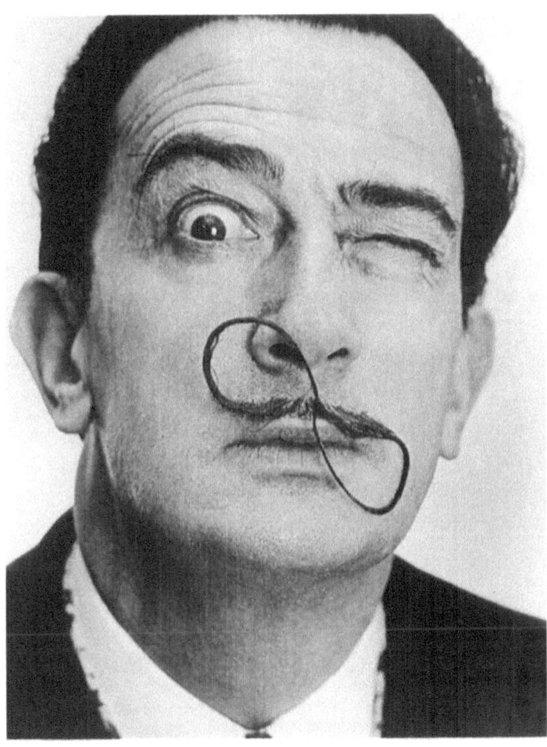

M.J. Johnson – If you want a modern day beard success story look no further than Minneapolis man M.J. Johnson. Johnson says he struggled to grow facial hair in High School and didn't even seriously decide to start growing his facial hair until he saw photos from the 2009 World Beard Championship. He may not be as famous as some of the others in this list, but there's no denying the epicness of his bear

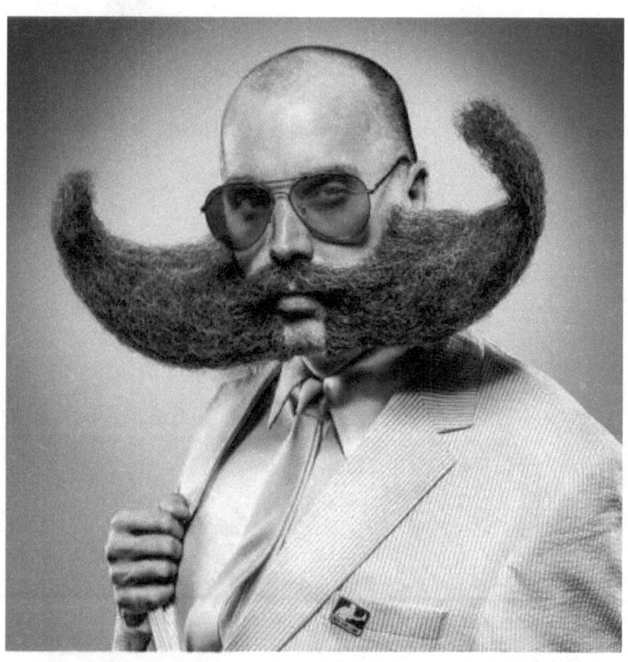

Figure 10 - M. J. Johnson. Just gonna let the picture stand on its own.

Kenny Rogers – say what you will about his music (I grew up with it, so of course I love it . . . but I get that it may be a taste some never acquire) there's no denying the power of Kenny's beard. If "The Coward of the County" had grown a beard like Roger's, he wouldn't have been called "Coward of the County". The beard just looks like it was MEANT to be on his face. In fact, ManBasics refuses to believe that Roger's wasn't in fact BORN with said beard until we see photographic evidence to the contrary. And even then, we will go full on conspiracy theory mode and claim the evidence is faked.

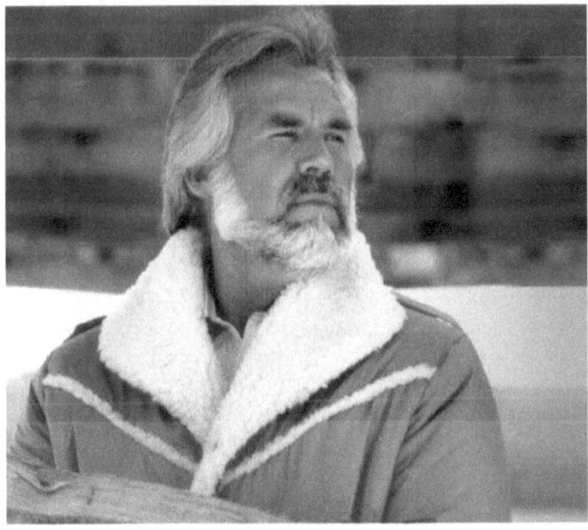

Figure 11 - Kenny Rogers makes us question our own beard.

Ron Swanson – OK, this one's another cheat . . . because it's more about Ron's moustache than his beard.   We included it because A) the moustache is epic and iconic, B) We love Ron Swanson and C) We love Ron Swanson. Did we mention we love Ron Swanson?

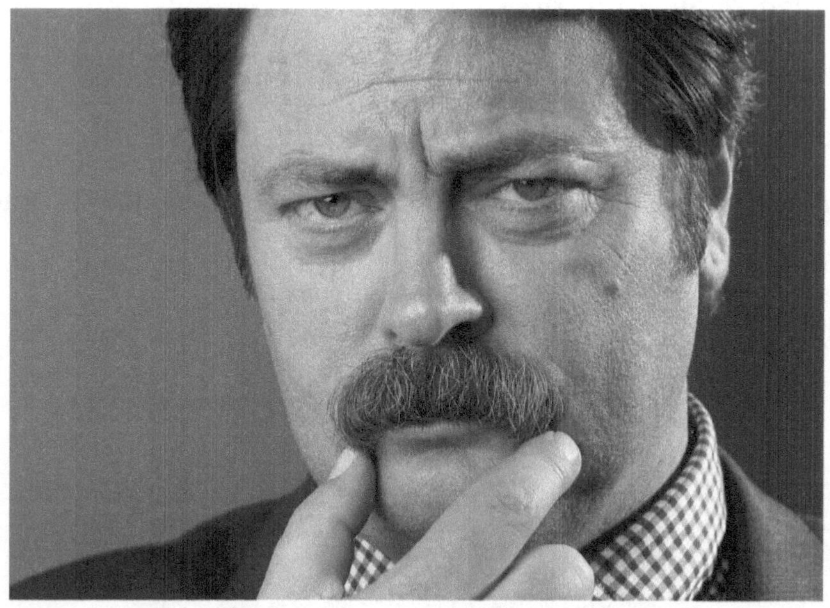

Figure 12 - Ron Swanson: "I'm a simple man. I like pretty, dark-haired women and breakfast food."

James Harden – "Home" for ManBasics is Houston, so we HAVE to give a shout out to James Harden who has a beard well known around the entire globe. I mean, his nickname is literally "The Beard", so you KNOW it's pretty epic. Harden has the distinction of having been the NBA 6th Man of the Year as WELL as becoming the league's MVP . . . which is definitely a testament to his dedication to always be getting better at his craft. We certainly think his beard just keeps getting better as well.

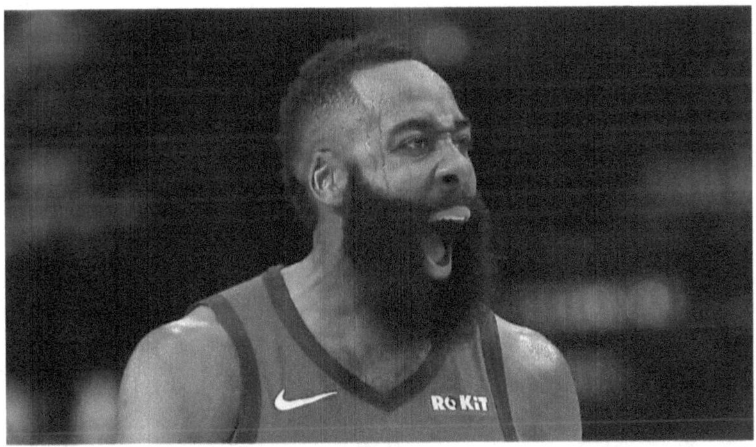

Figure 13 - James Harden is simply "The Beard.

Chapter Three – Why Even Grow A Beard?

First off, let's get one thing straight. You don't need a reason to grow a beard. I mean, that's part of the appeal of the beard in the first place, right? On some conscious or unconscious level you looked at societal norms (which is to say "shaving") and said "Forget that, I'm gonna do MY thing."

Now, that decision may have been as innocuous as simply growing a little Flavor Saver under your bottom lip, or going full-on Grizzly Adams, but the point is you decided to go against the norm.

And we may as well address the Elephant in the Barbershop…why IS shaving the societal norm in the first place? We went over the history a little bit already, and you will recall that having a beard WAS the status quo for several thousand years of human existence. How did we go from "Only the rich shave their beards" to "Only hippies and hipsters sport a chin curtain?"

After all, not only is growing a beard our natural state of being, religions have a surprising amount to say about beard growth.

Muslims believe Muhammed dictated: "Trim the moustache and leave the beard," which seems pretty clear. Sunnis believe this means trimming the beard is forbidden entirely, while the Shia believe that trimming of the beard is allowed. Complete shaving of the beard is believed by both to be "haram," which is to say "forbidden." So that means a little more than 42% of the world population believes that growing a beard is right and proper.

Judaism gets a little trickier. Leviticus 19:27 specifically states; "Do not cut the hair at the sides of your head or clip off the edges of your beard." That's also pretty straightforward, though it is in the same book of the Bible that bans unkempt hair, mixing fabrics in clothing, and getting tattoos.

Christianity is pretty well mum on the subject in the New Testament, but of course the Bible DOES include the Judaic Old Testament. However, 3rd Century Christian Teacher Clement of Alexandra deemed it impious "to desecrate the symbol of manhood, hairiness." Writing in 195 A.D., Clement also stated "But let the chin have the hair...for an ample beard suffices for men. And if one, too, must shave a part of his beard, it must not be made entirely bare, for this is a disgraceful sight." So Christianity seems to follow the all-or-nothing rule when it comes to beards.

Interesting.

Now to be clear, I don't want a bunch of strongly worded emails saying "Dude, you don't even know what that verse means...." and then going into a diatribe about religious interpretation. I'm not here to criticize any person or any religion or any religious practice, I'm just putting out there at face value (Hah!   I'm re-reading this while editing. See what I did there? "Face value"? Man . . . I'm good) what was (and is in many cases) believed based on the texts out there.

I'm throwing this all out there to show that in terms of society, there has historically been just as much pressure placed on a person to GROW a beard as there has been to NOT grow one. If that is true, how did we get where we are now?

Dare I say, where did we go wrong?

Like many things, there is no historical "aha!" moment. It just sort of gradually moved there. From what I can see, beards generally went in and out of style in the Western world based on the chin status of the King Du Jour. In America, our obsession with shaving is not dissimilar, mimicking the style of the President in power. It is no coincidence that some of the most epic beards in history are from the Civil War when the illustrious Abraham Lincoln sported epic locks. Ambrose Burnside, Robert E. Lee, James Longstreet…hell, just google "Civil War Generals" if you want to see a pretty epic display of amazing beards. There's not a clean-shaven gent among them other than Joseph Hooker (the term "hooker" is literally drawn from General Hooker, so I will just leave that little piece of beardless trivia there to stand on its own merits).

The last President to sport face fur was Benjamin Harrison from 1889 to 1893, and the last to have a moustache was William Howard Taft from 1909 to 1913. That means it has been over a hundred years since America has been led by someone with any facial hair at all. So as "trendy" as beards may appear currently, I think it is safe to say that America is currently in a "beards are out of style" phase. So to be clear, growing a beard is going against the grain. To be even more clear, that's a great reason in and of itself to grow one.

So returning to the question: why even grow a beard?

Here's the answer: you don't need a freaking reason. You do you, you beautiful bearded beast, you.

Chapter Four - Top Reasons Why You Should Grow A Healthy Beard

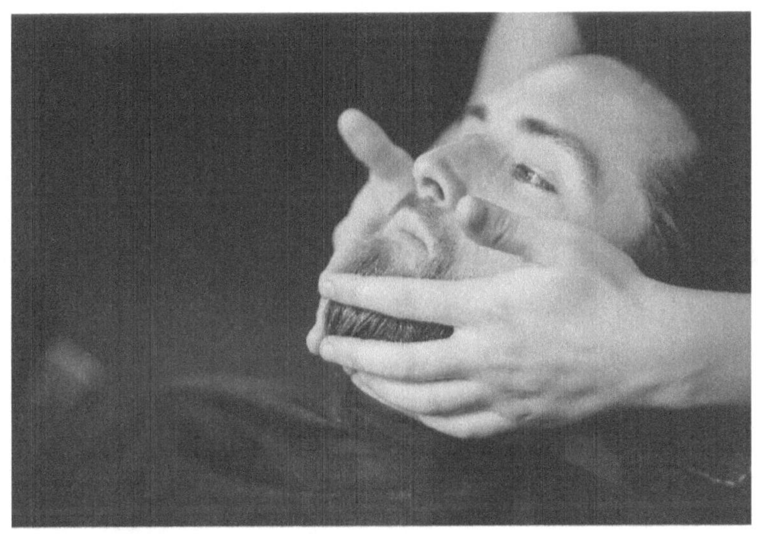

While you don't NEED a reason to grow a beard, there are plenty of great reasons to grow one, most of which have nothing to do with making you look totally kick ass. There are plenty of physical and even psychological benefits to tending your face foliage. Let's get into it!

1. Beards block Ultraviolet light

The results of a 2011 study published in the Journal Radiation Protection Dosimetry show that thick beards actually block a significant amount of ultraviolet sunlight (from 50-95%) from reaching the skin. This will protect your skin against sunburn as well as serve as a protection against getting skin cancer. The thicker the beard, the better it is at preventing UV light from getting through.

According to the University of Southern Queensland, four out of five cases of skin cancer in men occur on the face, head, or neck. "Facial hair has an Ultraviolet Protection Factor (UPF) of anywhere from 2 to 21," says Alfio Parisi, one of the study's authors and Professor of Radiation Physics at University of Southern Queensland in Toowoomba. A quality shirt has an SPF rating of 15, so a beard can literally be more protective to your face than a shirt is to your chest (and no, I didn't find any studies on how your chest hair effects SPF. If you have a hairy chest, go ahead and mentally give yourself a one point SPF bonus).

Certainly the thickness of your beard, the angle of the sun, the direct or indirect intensity of the sunlight are all factors at play here, but I think it is safe to say that a FaceFro is guaranteed to prevent face cancer (our lawyer insists that we point out the previous sentence was hyperbole).

2. It reduces infections

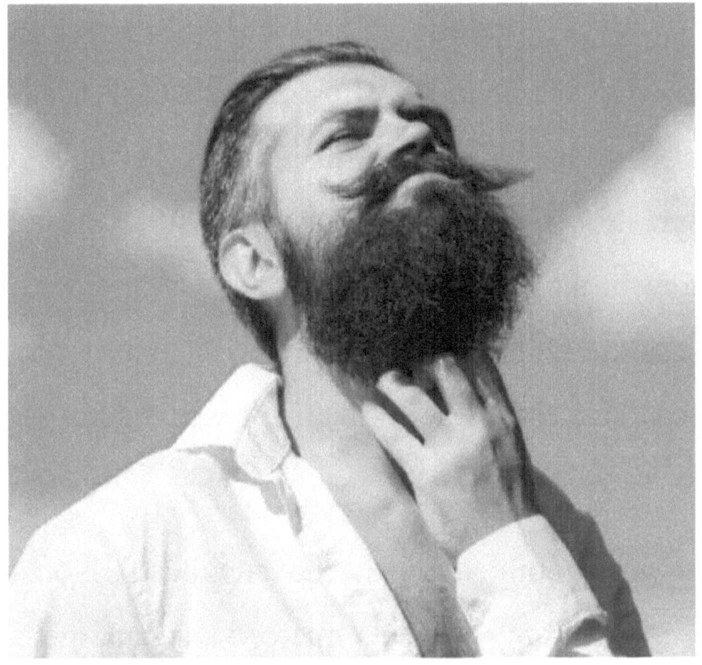

"I think that growing beard hair out can actually be helpful for some people," says University of Utah dermatologist Erika Summers, MD. "Irritant folliculitis, bacterial folliculitis and an inflammatory condition called pseudo folliculitis barbae can all occur in the beard area and are often precipitated by shaving." Many of these infections arise as a result of regular beard shaving. Understand that beards can also collect, trap, and grow bacteria if not tended to adequately. Proper beard hygiene is essential to your beard being a positive source of health and not a detriment.

Asthma patients or those who suffer from dust allergy or pollen can also benefit immensely from the reduced exposure to infection. The beard will filter the allergens and prevent them from having a field day on your body. It performs the same role as nasal hair in shutting unwanted allergens out from the skin. This will make you look healthier and stronger.

If you grow both a moustache and beard, you have a powerful tool to prevent microscopic allergens from turning your nose into a breeding ground for diseases. By keeping such allergens off your nose, you automatically have reduced chances of becoming infected with some allergens like hay and others.

This implies that a beard goes beyond just a fashion accessory. It can mean the difference between illness and good health. That could be a lifesaver when you least expect it. Obviously, it offers tons of health benefits that were previously unknown.

3. It helps keep your skin moist

Shaving naturally exposes your skin to dryness as the pores are unusually opened up and left without any protection. During the winter and summer, such exposed pores offer the perfect condition for moisture loss; a condition that can cause your skin to flake.

You guessed it, wearing a beautiful thick Dumbledore greatly reduces the possibility for these conditions. The skin is naturally prevented from dryness as the beard forms a protective layer around your face. Why Donald Trump doesn't have a beard is beyond me, as your beard will effectively "build the wall" around the sin on your face. As the beard keeps cold air and wind out of your face, it is easier for your skin to successfully overcome dryness.

Additionally, your beard enables the sebaceous glands (oil glands for short) to keep the moisture in your skin since it becomes nearly impossible for the moisture to dry out through the beard. According to Dr. Shannon C. Trotter, a fellow of the Osteopathic College of Dermatology, your beard literally secretes a natural oil that keeps skin moisturized. Well-moisturized skin will keep your face healthy and attractive.

4. You will have blemish-free skin

Shaving can do much damage to your skin without noticing it. Apart from exposing the pores in your skin, it also exposes you to cuts and other issues that will give you spots on your face. Razor rash, acne, and folliculitis (hair-follicle inflammation) are often the result of shaving,

However, when you don't shave and keep your beard in good shape, you greatly increase the chances of blemish free skin. Please note, this is with proper beard care and maintenance. More on this later.

5. Your beard: The Allergen Bouncer

We all know from sixth-grade health class that your nose hairs act as a filtration system that prevents dust, allergens, and pretty much anything airborne from getting into your body unwanted (remember, that's where "boogers" come from/ We can't believe it took this long in the book before we mentioned "boogers").

Well, what is a beard and mustache if not a GIANT air filtration system right under your nose? Your Chewbacca face is like that big-ass bouncer at the club and allergens are that annoying punk who tries to cut in line and talk his way into the club.

Thankfully your beard is there to say "I'm afraid I don't see your name on the list sir".

According to Dr. Clifford W. Bassett, Allergy and Asthma Care of NY medical director, the more hair you have under your airways (read: the bigger your beard), the more pollutants you're snaring every day.

Keep in mind that like any filter, it needs to be cleaned regularly in order to stay effective and sanitary. If you aren't exercising good beard hygiene then you are basically KEEPING all those allergens you trapped…which is decidedly defeating the purpose. More on maintaining a clean Chin Curtain to come of course.

6. Manliness power up

The Journal of Evolution and Human Behavior actually did a study in 2013 on how women (AND men) perceive people with beards. Spoiler alert: men with beards were perceived as more masculine than men with a smooth face. But as bearded brethren, we both knew that instinctively, am I right?

A 2008 study in Psychology Today determined that women find men with beards as " masculine, aggressive, and socially mature." They also believe beards made men look older, which depending on age may or may not be a good thing.   Furthermore (and certainly interestingly), women rated men with full beards as highest for perceived parenting ability and healthiness. Presumably the photos women were looking at did not include Rasputin or Tywin Lannister.

So, it's no wonder that growing a beard has the potential to give you a confidence boost. We are basically hard wired to dig people with beards. It's like getting that Power Up in a video, but this power up is for "Manliness."

Chapter Five - Maintain That Kick-Ass Beard – A Beard Regimen

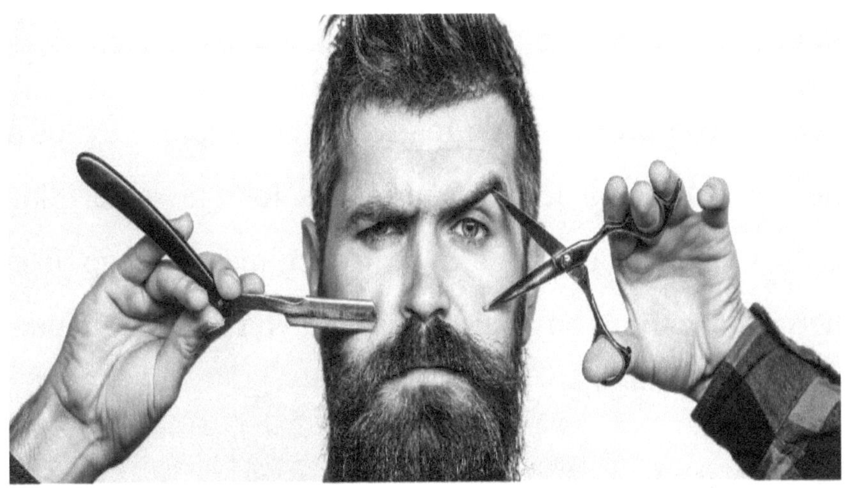

For men that like to look manly, but not like wooly wildebeests, there are a number of great products on the market to help a brother out. So you want to look classy, fashion-conscious and attractive? I'll tell you which products will help you up your game and take your overall appearance as seriously as possible.

Navigating the wide variety of beard products can actually be a little daunting. Beard oil? Beard Balm? Beard

Conditioner?   Beard Butter?   Do I need some of these?
All of these?   None of these?

Add to the mix product hardware like beard trimmers and
electric razors, beard comb, beard brushes, straighteners . .
. it begins to look like a giant hairy jungle out there.

Take a deep breath.   It's really pretty simple.   A lot of
these are different terms or products for the same thing.
Let's start with a standard beard regimen and go from
there. Depending on your beard style you may not include
everything listed here.   Let's dig in:

1.   **Wash it**

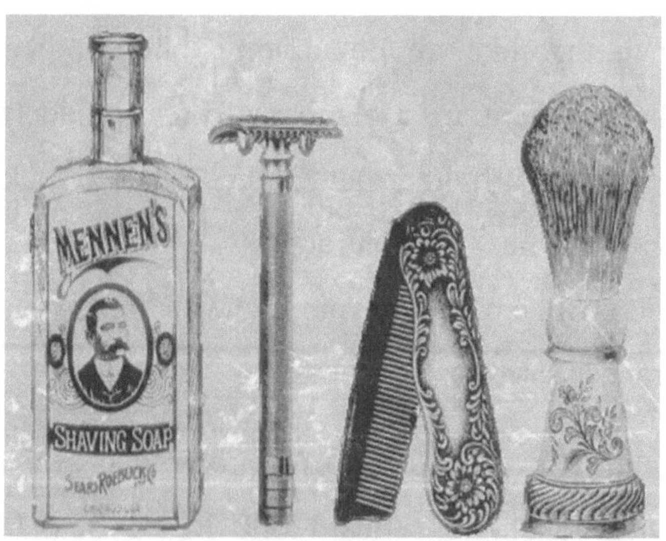

A recent study conducted by *European Radiology* suggested that men with beards had higher amounts of bacteria than dogs. Dafuq?

Guys, this is fine. Really.

As mentioned before, your beard is basically a giant filter that is enhancing and doing similar work as the hairs found in your nostrils. It makes complete sense that you would find increased levels of bacteria and germs in your beard. It means those germs and bacteria never made it into your mouth or nose! Your beard has fulfilled its function (other than making you look totally kickass).

That said, you still have a beard full of bacteria, germs and allergens! You gotta wash that shit.

Don't wash your beard with just regular soap, especially store bought bar soap which will dry your skin out. Rather, you can get some beard-specific soaps or shampoos that will soften the beard and prevent it from drying out. Most face washes are designed for your face, not for just any hair, so a beard-specific wash is definitely recommended, but perfect is the enemy of good. A liquid face wash is way better than bar soap.

Apart from a beard-specific beard wash, we would only suggest washing your beard two or three times a week max unless you have a conditioning regimen. You should still wash your face daily, but your body is already producing oils to help your beard naturally stay healthy. Daily beard washing will strip those oils out of your beard. If you get your beard dirty by playing a pick-me-up game of basketball or working on your brother-in-law's '79 Camaro, then by all means give it another wash. You CAN wash it daily but only if you plan to maintain your beard further (more on that next).

If you don't have a beard wash then use a mild soap, preferably a liquid soap which tends to be gentler than bar soap. Remember, the goal here is to clean well enough to remove unwanted bacteria while also not being so harsh as to remove the natural oils in your beard. A mild shampoo can be a good backup here if you don't have a wash designed for beards. But remember, shampoo is designed for *head hair* and can leave your skin dry. Bar soaps are designed for *body skin*, which can leave your beard and face dry. That is why we highly recommend finding an appropriate beard wash. It's the Goldilocks of beard cleaning …it needs to be *just right.*

This perfect blend solution is essentially going to be both a "wash" AND A "conditioner." It will gently wash your beard while also restoring the natural oils and sebum it would otherwise be stripping out. Of course, we recommend the ManBasics "Not Your Girlfriends Beard Wash for this purpose!

Summing up: Listen to your beard . . . and face. If you are washing your face every day and getting dry skin, flaky skin, or dandruff then try to only wash it every couple days, especially if you don't have a proper beard wash. We highly suggest getting a beard wash designed for beards, which will give you the freedom to wash it daily and really keep your beard hygienic and healthy.

Regardless, you are going to want to condition your beard, ESPECIALLY on days you have washed it.

After your shower, go ahead and just towel dry your beard and move on to conditioning.

2. Condition the Beard

What do you normally do after you wash your hair?   You put conditioner in it. That's because the shampoo process not only cleans out the dirt and filth that was in your hair, but ALSO strips out the natural oils (sebum) in your hair.

What do most of us do after washing our face and beard? Probably nothing.

Conditioning your beard is basically putting back IN the natural oils that you already took OUT in the washing process. It is VERY important in order to not dry out your skin.

Growing a beard is great for you in a LOT of ways, but keeping your face moist isn't one of them. Facial hair draws up a lot of the moisture in your face skin from the surface where it evaporates quickly. This, in turn, leaves the skin underneath dry and flaky.

In other words, your beard is like a plant and your face is watering it, so we need to make sure our face has plenty of moisture to provide your beard. Not enough moisture and your face will dry out and well . . . die. That's what dry skin and flakes are, right? Dead skin falling off your face. Don't murder your face bro, moisturize it.

There are tons of different terms for beard conditioners: Beard Oil, Beard Balm, Beard Butter, Beard Wax, Beard Conditioner, Leave-in Conditioner . . . all of these serve the same function of moisturizing your face and your beard. The next chapter will go in to the difference between all these products so you can chose the one that makes the most sense for you and your beard.

All of these conditioning products should have an easy reading ingredient list. You are putting natural oils back into your hair, not strange chemicals you have never heard of before. We don't want to be too "crunchy" here, but if your conditioner is full of ingredients you can't pronounce, it is likely not a high-quality product. (Shameless plus here . . . at <u>ManBasics</u> we like to say we leave out the harsh chemicals and stick to the basics: ManBasics. Pretty catchy, huh?).

Your beard shampoo will likely have a few unusual terms, because a shampoo will be a mix of ingredients that 1) won't naturally bind together and as such 2) will need a preservative to be shelf stable and not grow the very bacteria it is meant to cleanse.

Not so with a beard oil or beard balm. All the ingredients can and should work well together. Some of the best benefits of a quality conditioning product will be inherent to the ingredients themselves. There is also no need for perfume, parfum, scents, or fragrances either. Great scent will be derived from essential oils, which have their own specific benefits AND smell great.

3. Brush the beard regularly

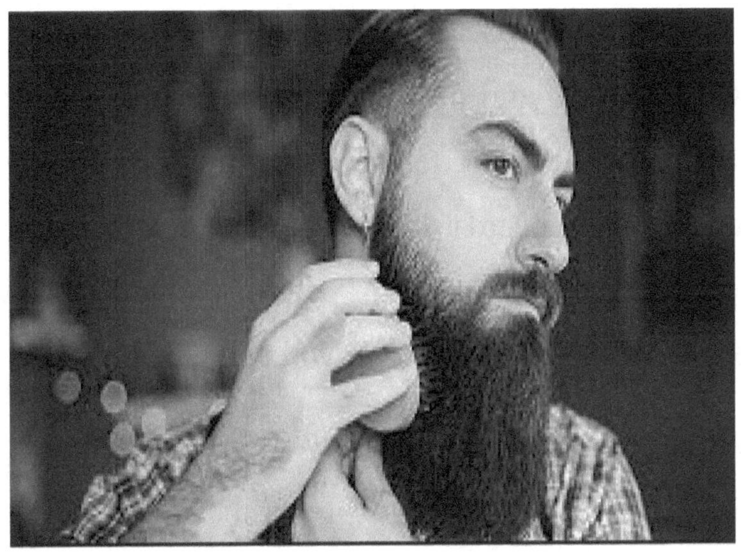

Combing and or brushing your beard serves several purposes. For longer beards it will help to remove and prevent tangles. For beards of any length it will help to train the beard to grow straight (not unlike your pubes or underarm hair, it will want to naturally curl without encouragement otherwise). The longer your beard grows the more important it will be to use a comb and/ or brush to help keep your beard styled. Styling your beard not only makes it look great, but helps to prevent ingrown hairs. Also, a good beard brush will lightly exfoliate your skin as brushing your beard effectively is brushing the skin on your face as well.

The main difference in use between a comb and a brush will likely be your beard length. In general, a beard brush will be used for shorter beards, while a comb is ideal for longer length beards. If you begin using a beard brush but feel like you are merely "petting" your beard with the brush, it is likely time to get yourself a comb.

What to look for in a brush – Certainly some of this will be subjective in terms of aesthetics and ergonomic preferences. At <u>ManBasics</u>, we like the look and feel of an all-natural wood brush, but there is no real reason a plastic handle brush can't work just as well for you, especially if you like the way it fits in your hand better than some other brand of brush.

What we WILL suggest though is that you get a brush made with genuine boar hair or horsehair. Like many things in this world, God and nature got it right in the original design. Natural hair fibers are ideal for both brushing your hair and evenly distributing any oils, balms, or conditioners you have put into your beard. We think boar bristles are ideal because they have the perfect amount of stiffness to style your beard while not damaging or tearing at your hair like stiff nylon bristles tend to do. Horse hair is a little softer and will more likely brush OVER your hair instead of through it.

What to Look for in a Comb - For your comb, the biggest concern here is what the comb is made of (other than the aforementioned aesthetic and ergonomic concerns). There are plenty of cheap combs out there. Don't fall for them.

Cheap plastic combs can actually tear at your beard hairs with microscopic splits in the comb caused by mass machinery manufacture. These tiny imperfections will grab on to your beard and pull at them like your ex-girlfriend when she showed up at happy hour begging you to take her back and wouldn't let you go. It wasn't pretty. Also like your ex, it just isn't very good for you (or your beard).

Our material of choice here is sandalwood. Sandalwood combs LOOK great but have other advantages as well. First, sandalwood is a material that will be found in many beard oils and balms in the form of an essential oil. The wood mixed with the oils smell great.

It also does a great job of working through your hair to detangle and style your beard effectively. The denseness of the wood will act as a natural massage on your face. Seriously, using a sandalwood comb makes beard care a luxury instead of a chore each day. There's a reason that sandalwood combs are the most popular option in the beard community.

Another good option is ox horn, if only because it sounds badass to be combing your beard with ox horn. It is also known to be anti-static, so your beard won't have any weird static cling.

In terms of teeth size there are a lot of options out there. Obviously the wider the bristles the easier it is to go through your beard and the less actual "combing" there is to do. Our preference is to use a double-sided comb, which has a "rough comb" on one side and a "fine comb" on the other. This gives you the flexibility to work on nearly any beard size and length.

Lastly, a beard COMB can be a great "assistant" during the beard trimming process, which is a great segue way to . . .

4. Trim the beard

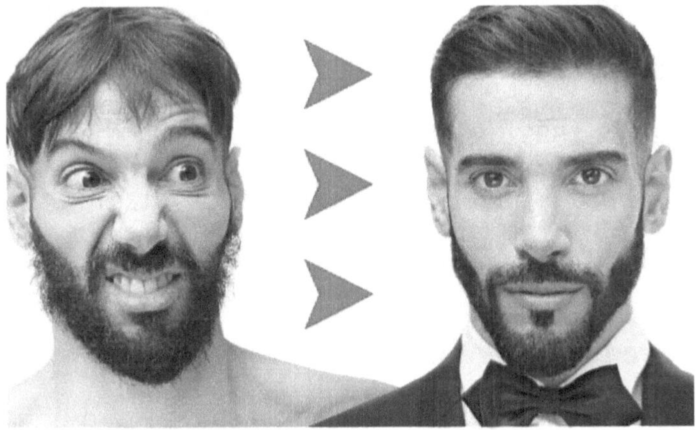

After conditioning and brushing your beard is the perfect time to give it a trim if needed. We'll have more detail on the mechanics of shaping your beard, but the basics of simply trimming it and keeping it relatively even are pretty simple.

One technique we like to use goes against the grain…literally. Take your beard comb and brush against the grain of your beard. This will make the hairs stand up and out, making it easier to use the trimmer as well as enabling you to see wild growing hairs more easily.

Run the electric trimmer through your beard, working against the grain like you did with the comb. For God's sake, err on the side of using too high a number on your trimmer guard. There's nothing more tragic than a man accidentally shaving off more of his beard than he meant to (OK, there probably ARE some more tragic things, but allow us a little hyperbole here).

If you aren't seeing any difference (or seeing any hair in your sink), switch to a lower number. You will have made some decisions about what kind of beard you are trying to shape, but a pretty common method is to have a "two guard" difference between your chin and your sideburns: for example, a five length on your chin and a three length for your sideburns.

Lastly, don't forget the final crucial step of actually shaving. If you are not going for the "wild unkempt" look, then sadly, shaving is still a part of your daily grooming, just in a lesser fashion.

Shaving your lower neckline is important for your overall look: get too close to your jawline and it will look like you have a double chin. Too far down and you look like a mountain man. Most people go for a line just above your Adam's apple.

Look at yourself in the mirror and find the center point above your Adam's apple. Visualize an imaginary curved line going from there to behind each ear. This is your trimline. Err on the side of going below this line at first, as you can always shave a little more but can't "un-shave" if you go too high. Afterwards, rub a little beard oil in as it is a great skin moisturizer in addition to being great for your beard.

Oh, and brush your beard back in place if you haven't already.

Now, a word about clippers. They come in all shapes and sizes with a wide variety of bells and whistles. For the most part, this really is a matter of personal preference. Here are a few of the major options to consider:

- Wired or Cordless – My preference is to go cordless, but it can be frustrating if you have a trimmer that is not charged and ready to go at all times.

- Quality – Better trimmers will be made with stainless steel blades. There will be a wide variety of price and quality options out there. But we suggest not skimping on the stainless steel, otherwise you will be buying another one a few months later.

- Length Options – Most trimmers will have guard attachments to handle the beard length adjustments you want. Some trimmers will have adjustable length on the trimmer itself. This really is a matter of preference and also where some of the wide variety of pricing options present themselves. If your needs are simple, you can save a few bucks by having fewer options here.

- Dry Trimming or Wet Trimming – Some trimmers will be waterproof, which is certainly convenient if you like to do your trimming in the shower. Personally, I don't have a mirror in the shower and I prefer to see what I am doing.

- Bells and Whistles – Some will have some weird options, like a vacuum that sucks up the trimmed hairs as you are trimming. For me, less is more but if you gotta have the trimmer with built-in Bluetooth speakers that doubles as an egg poacher, hey…the heart wants what the heart wants.

5. **Shape the beard (optional)**

   Depending on your beard or moustache look you are going for this may be an optional step. This would be when you add in beard or moustache wax and use it to literally "shape" your beard.

   No, Salvadore Dali's moustache didn't just "grow" like that, and neither will yours. Wax is used to practically glue your hair to a specific shape. There are lots of different balms and waxes out there, and they will really come down to your personal preference on how much "hold" they have.

One thing that nearly all beard brothers might consider though is a little bit of shaping with a beard butter or balm. I like to add a little beard balm to my palm and just rub over my beard once. This can help with any hair "fly aways".

Chapter Six – Beard Conditioners

So, we have already mentioned in the last chapter that there are a wide variety of "Beard Conditioners". Each has their own properties and uses, some of which are overlapping. In theory, you can be completely extra and use several or all of these options. More likely, you will pick a beard regimen that works for you and matches your lifestyle and beard/face chemistry.

Why Use Beard Conditioners

I know we have already discussed this issue previously, but we cannot stress enough how important it is to condition your beard on a regular basis. How often you condition will have to do with how active you are (which likely determines how often you wash your beard), what sort of cleansing products you are using, and simple genetics which determine whether you have a naturally oily complexion or a dry one.

A common complaint within the community of beard growers is dry, flaky, or itchy skin . . . even amongst people who normally don't have skin issues. So it would appear that the dryness is a derivative of the beard or beard growing process itself.

And it is.

Think of your beard as a vegetable garden. Now, you want your vegetables to be nice and healthy so of course you want your tomatoes and jalapenos and eggplants to get plenty of water and fertilizer. So, naturally you put plenty of water and fertilizer onto the tomatoes, jalapenos and eggplant right?

Wrong.

I mean, you may water the veggies incidentally, but you are watering THE GROUND. You are placing the fertilizer on THE SOIL.

That's because plants ingest their nutrients through their roots . . . which are in the ground. If you want big juicy tomatoes you tend the soil as much or even more than the vegetables themselves.

I'm sure you figured this out already . . . but your beard is the veggies and the soil is your face (sorry guys, I understand this metaphor would have been more kick-ass if I had figured out a way to incorporate "bacon" instead of "veggies". We're gonna go cook some bacon right now as penance and give a salad the stink eye at lunch today on general principal).

Always remember that a healthy beard begins with healthy facial care. Healthy facial care begins with watering and fertilizing your face by moisturizing it with a variety of conditioners, beginning with beard oil.

Beard Oils

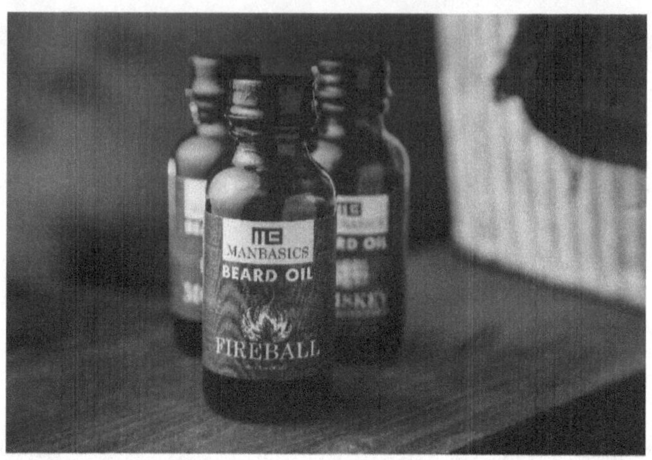

Figure 14 - <u>High quality beard oils</u> are an essential tool to maintain a healthy beard

Beard oils are probably the easiest to find and most common beard conditioner. Beard oil is exactly what it sounds like: oils that you apply to your beard in order to replace the oils in your beard and face that you washed out when washing your face and beard.

This is THE core element of good beard care, because it is a liquid that will easily apply to you face as well as your beard as you are rubbing it in.

Beard oils should be made up of two basic components: carrier oils and scent oils. The scent oils will be either essential oils, or fragrance oils

Essential Oils – Essential oils will make up a very small percentage of your beard oil, likely only 1-2% of the total blend. That's because essential oils are exactly what they sound like, the concentrated "essence" of the plant material they represent.

As you can imagine, these oils are so concentrated that they actually need to be seriously diluted to prevent them from actually doing more harm than good to your beard or face.

Essential oils are the ultimate in home remedy, homeopathic, apothecary, medicine man solutions. There is PLENTY of evidence that essential oils can and do have medicinal and therapeutic benefits.   At <u>ManBasics</u>, we like to take claims with a grain of salt . . . while also recognizing that boatloads of modern medicine is built oin the shoulders of herbal remedies, if not being outright lab created copies of said herbs.

So we take it seriously when we find studies that show certain essential oils have benefits to you skin or hair.

Please seen our appendix for a list of some of our favorite essential oils that aid in beard and face skin care.

Plus, they simply smell good as well.

Fragrance Oils – Fragrance oils are similar to essential oils in scent only. They are basically lab created concoctions created to emulate the scent (fragrance) of an essential oil, or perhaps a scent that doesn't exist at all as an essential oil.

Fragrance oils have gotten a lot of press of late as being potentially dangerous ingredients. The problem people have with fragrance oils is that they are such a small percentage of the ingredient pool that it is not required by the FDA to disclose specific ingredients it contains.

As such, it's really hard to say specifically what IS in a beard oil that says "fragrance oil" or simply "fragrance". It could be something perfectly innocuous, it could be something very dangerous, or it could be something that is just not very good for YOU specifically, because you have an allergy to a specific ingredient that has not been disclosed.

That's why at <u>ManBasics</u> we opt to use essential oils over fragrance oils in nearly every case. At the end of the day you have three choices:

1) Essential oils that smell good and have a long history of proven benefits to your body
2) Fragrance oils that smell good but provide no benefits to your beard and face
3) Fragrance oils that smell good but are actually bad for you

I think you can see why we err on the side of essential oils . . . all the upside and no downside (unless you have an essential oil allergen . . . and yeah, that can be a thing).

Carrier Oils – Carrier oils will make up 98-99% of your beard oil. As we mentioned, essential oils need to be diluted and fragrance oils are crafted to emulate the same scent strength of essential oils.

There are plenty of oils that will qualify as a quality carrier oil, some as common as olive oil or almond oil. Most all oils will have some specific benefits to you beard and face, so it really comes down to finding an oil that has the ingredients with not only benefits to your face and beard, but also to the scent and feel of the oil itself. Consult our appendix for a list of carrier oil benefits.

Basically, beard oils will be the foundation of your beard and face conditioning process. We recommend you put a few drops of beard oil in your hand after taking a shower and drying your beard. Rub it between your palm to warm it up and then rub it into your beard.

You are striving to not only coat your beard but your face as well. Remember, your face is feeding moisture to your beard so you need to feed moisture to your face. If you have a big beard you will want to apply a little more, and you will likely use a beard balm or butter as well.

Beard Butters, Balms, and Waxes

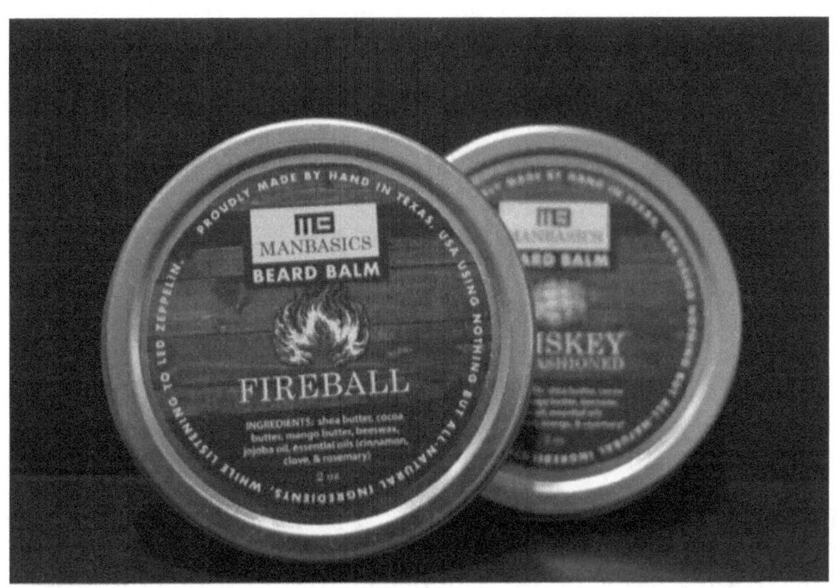

Butters, balms and waxes are all sides of the same coin (well, if you had a coin with three sides). All of these products take the basics of a beard oil but add a variety of butters and waxes which have different moisturizing benefits to your basic beard oil, and will ALSO add some measure of "hold" to your beard.

As a maker of all-natural products, for ManBasics the difference between these three products would be summed up in the amount of beeswax we add to a recipe. A butter would have the least amount of beeswax and have (spoiler alert) a "buttery" consistency to it. The amount of hold would be more than an oil, which provides almost no hold at all, but certainly wouldn't shape your beard into unnatural positions. Basically, it could be used to give a once over on your beard and prevent any stray hairs from flying away.

A "balm" will have more beeswax and provide more hold a shaping ability. Again, it likely won't hold your beard in any radically unusual positions, but it will most likely be able to give your beard a general direction or help gravity in keeping your hair staying down.

Beard Wax as its name implies will have the most amount of wax. When you see beard and moustaches like M.J. Johnson or Salvadore Dali, you are looking at high wax content product.

So, as you move up the scale from butters to balms to wax, the percentage of wax (typically beeswax) increases. Beeswax doesn't do nearly as much for your beard as oils and butters, so the less "moisturizing" your product is doing. So, if you are dealing with dry skin you might want to sacrifice shaping ability for moisturizing ability.

That brings us to the ability of a balm and butter to moisturize your beard. In short, it's amazing. First, the butters themselves have nearly all the same moisturizing benefits of beard oils. See our appendix for some of our favorite butters and their benefits.

Butters, balms and waxes all ALSO include actual beard carrier oils IN the product in addition to the butters. Because of the higher viscosity of the butters, a beard balm or butter will sit on your beard longer, delivering more of a "slow release" of moisturizing benefits, as opposed to a beard oil which gets absorbed into your skin and beard almost immediately.

So, if you are battling dandruff, dry skin, or itchy skin and a beard oil alone is not helping you really should consider trying a high-quality beard balm or beard butter. If you apply beard oil in moderation you can even use BOTH products. In fact, at ManBasics we tend to put a beard oil in, groom and brush our beard, then hit it last with a little bit of beard balm to help keep the fly aways down and extra condition our beard.

One more things about beard butters, balms and waxes – it's important to check that ingredient list. There's really no need for these products to have a long list of complicated ingredients. Butters, oils, wax, essential oils or fragrance are as complicated as it should be.

If you see a bunch of unpronounceable words, or ingredients with numbers in them . . . these are dead giveaways that the manufacturer if using chemicals with questionable benefits at best and downright harmful consequences at worst.

We won't mention names, but one beard balm manufacturer (who you would know if you heard their trademark whistle) produces a beard balm with a long list of unfamiliar ingredients . . . including methylparaben. Parabens are potential endocrine disruptors due to their ability to mimic estrogen.

So to be clear . . . this unnamed company is making a manly product (does it GET more manly than making a beard balm?) that has ingredients mimicking . . . ESTROGEN? Dafuq?

As we mentioned before, at ManBasics we like to stick to the basics whenever we can. We have a few products that by their nature require a preservative of some kind in order to be shelf stable . . . but beard oils and beard balms don't have any water. There's no reason you can't find cost effective all natural products here and we strongly suggest you use them.

Beard Conditioner

So, here is where things get wonky. Beard oils, beard balms, and beard butters are all synonyms for "beard conditioner", but none of them look like what we traditionally think of as a "hair conditioner". So, when you are googling "beard conditioner" you will find beard oils and balms etc, but may ALSO find something that is more like a traditional "lotion" conditioner that we are used to using in the shower.

Basically, this category of product can be a little all over the place. We think there are some great products here, but to try and give a general rule for what these are and how they should be used would be a losing battle. There are some self described beard conditioners meant to be used and washed out in the shower like a head hair conditioner, there are others that function like a beard oil or balm and put in post shower.

Basically, we highly recommend you read the manufacturers instructions (and ingredients!) to learn what you are dealing with. Lotion type conditioners could be a little more complicated in their ingredients list, as they could contain ingredients like water which necessitate having a preservative. This won't necessarily be a bad thing, but it will definitely be a more complicated ingredient list than an all-natural beard oil.

One interesting subset of beard conditioners is an overnight leave in conditioner. This will basically be a conditioner meant to be left in overnight so that it moisturizes while you sleep. Sweet!

Basically, you are looking for a product that will release its moisturizing benefits slowly, like a beard balm or butter does. There will be some "lotion" style products in this as well, but the general idea is the same.

At <u>ManBasics</u> we started using a leave in conditioner with fantastic results. After a month of using we found our beards NOTICEABLY softer than when we started. Guys, if your ladies are complaining about your beard being too stiff or scratchy, then a leave in conditioner is the way to go. At ManBasics we rub some of our <u>Unscented Overnight Beard Balm</u> blend into our beard before we turn in. We like to use products that are more gently or completely unscented here as it can be difficult to fall asleep with strong scents emanating from right under your nose.

Chapter Seven – Beard Shapes and Styles

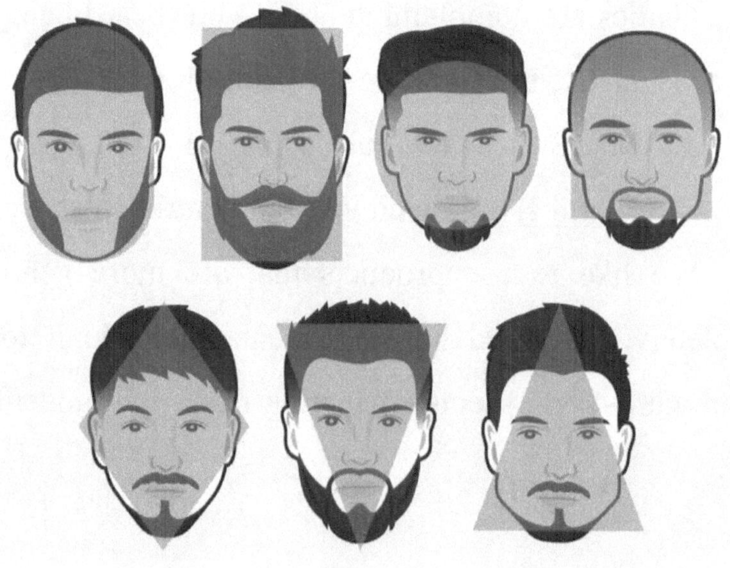

Now here's where things start getting fun! You get to decide what style and shape of beard you want, and believe me, there are more styles than you'd think. They range anywhere from Three Musketeers dandy to burly Mountain Man, to rogueish devil. These actually have names. Let's go over them, shall we?

The full beard – This one's so manly it could be considered the father of all beards. It's the classic, combining sideburns, a mustache, AND a beard for a full show of rugged manliness. So long as it's kept trimmed and oiled, this style of beard is perfect for any occasion. It says "ready for anything" without making a big fuss or show about it.

The Balbo – This is a more cultivated-looking beard, styled with intention. You could call it a dandy's beard, with a chinstrap, a soul patch, and a handlebar mustache. For whatever reason, it's a requirement with the that the beard never touch the mustache. Plenty of facial coverage with this one, if you're into that.

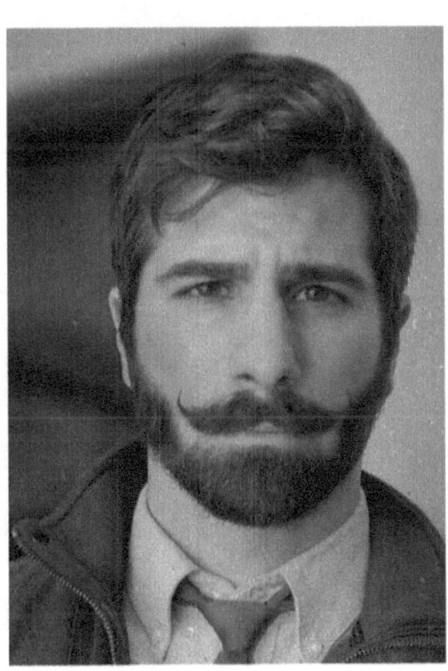

Figure 15 - A Balbo Beard with Stylin' 'Stache

Mutton Chops beard – Another classic style, this man fur style consists of long, full sideburns that connect to a mustache, but usually without any hair on the chin. This style is well-suited to guys with rounder faces. This one got its name because of its resemblance to the actual mutton chop---so you know a beard named after a hunk of meat is a good way to go.

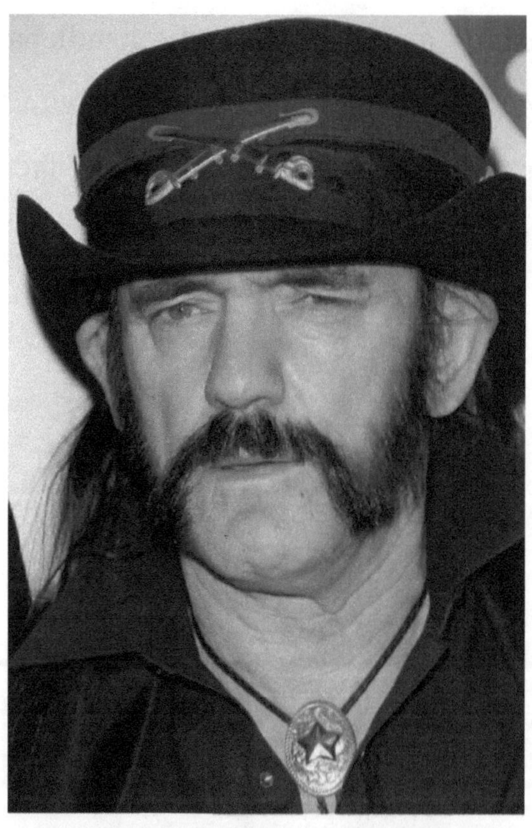

Figure 16 - Rocker Lemmy rocks a classic mutton chop.

Van Dyke beard – This is a type of goatee where the chin hair is disconnected from the mustache hair. For extra flair, some men like to wing out the ends of the moustache like a handlebar, and then pull the chin hair down into a narrow point. It's fancy!

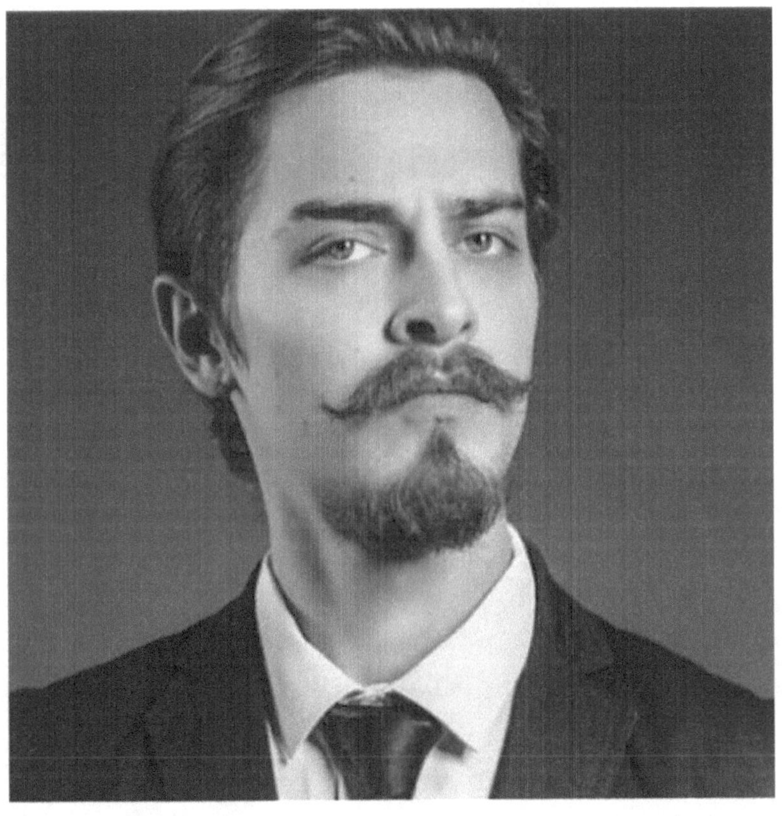

Figure 17 - The Classic Van Dyke.   Oh we fancy.

The goatee – Most dudes flirt with the idea of growing a beard by trying a goatee first. The opposite of the fully-committed mutton chop style in a way…this style features hair ONLY on the chin. It can be worn many different ways, narrow, or full—sometimes it's called a "goat patch" or a "chin puff."

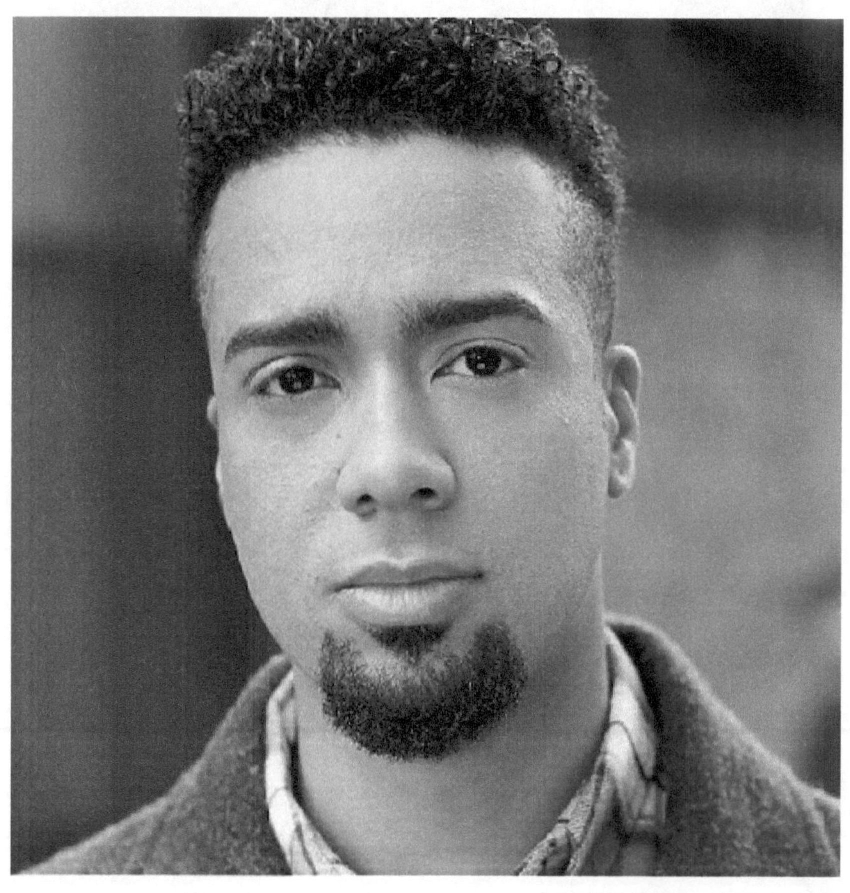

Figure 18 - The Goatee, just a little chin music.

Chinstrap beard – Much like it sounds, the chinstrap style only has hair around the lower jaw, running from sideburn to sideburn. It does not extend up into a moustache or grow on the cheeks. It's thus named because it resembles a helmet strap attached to one's chin.

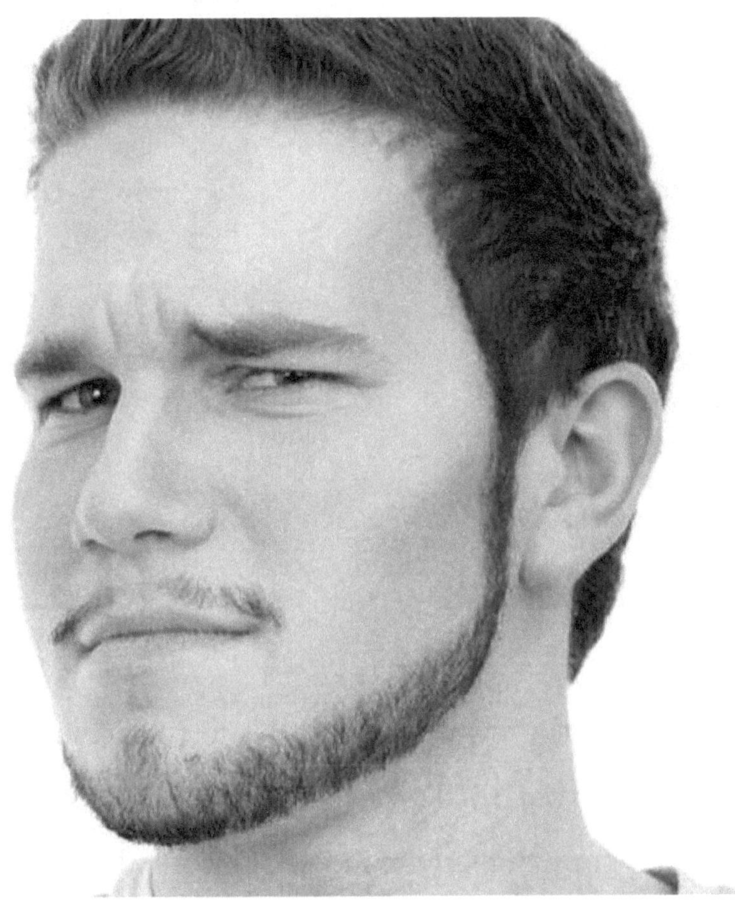

Figure 19 - Chinstrap Beard nice and tight.

Gunslinger beard – For dudes who don't mind being called cowpoke, podnah, or buckaroo…this beard hearkens back to Old West style. It has flared sideburns paired with a horseshoe moustache.

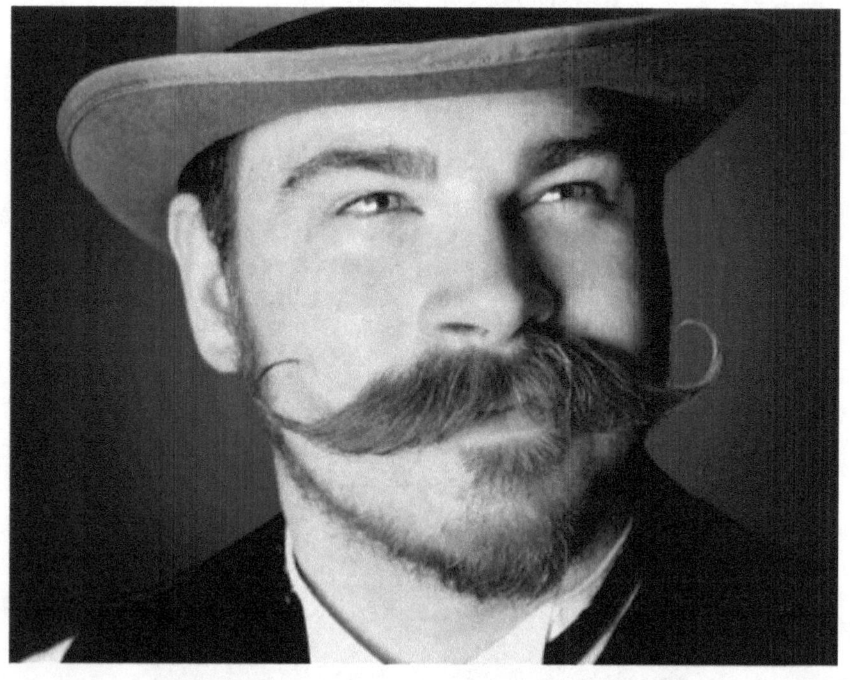

Figure 20 - The Gunslinger, always a classic.

These are just a few different styles to consider….there are many more, but I'll leave that to you to discover as you explore your potential bearddom. One good way to choose your future beard style is to consider the shape of your face.

If you have an oblong or rectangular face, try out a full beard, chin curtain, or chin strap beard. Rounder faces do well with some chop styles, a soul patch, goatee, anchor, or royale beard because they all add some angles to the face. An oval or inverted triangle shape face would look great in mutton chops, extended goatee, or even just some designer stubble.

Whatever shape face you have there's a perfect beard style out there, just waiting to decorate it.

Chapter Ten - Let's Get Extra

This chapter will basically be a few odds and ends that I couldn't figure out where else to put them. So here's a few random shots.

Beard Straighteners – Most guys beards are pretty naturally curly. Like . . . pubic hair curly. Now, there are some out there who turn their nose up at the idea of even bothering to try and straighten out your beard. The argument here is that you are "cheating" by making your beard look longer than it actually is.

While we certainly can respect this minimalist point of view, we also recognize that all beards are beautiful, and they come in a wide variety of styles. Some of these styles are gonna require a little help, and that's where we come to beard straighteners. If that's cheating, well . . . at ManBasics we use one, so I guess we're cheaters.

Beard straighteners are a relatively new phenomena in the beard world, but the idea of straightening your beard is not. Basically, a beard straightener is attempting to more efficiently replace using a hair dryer to accomplish the same effect. Allow us to explain.

ANY kind of heat will make your hair more malleable. A hair dryer, flat iron, beard straightener: the heat it produces breaks down your hair's hydrogen bonds, stripping away its natural oils and proteins. The heat changes your hair's texture, allowing you to mold it to create the look you want.

A beard straightener is basically a heated comb, which is much easier to use than a hair dryer or flat iron.

Now, please note what was stated above that this additional heat CAN damage your hair. It's important to put some product in your beard before using a beard straightener. Argan oil has a very high smoke point (420 degrees Fahrenheit/220 Celsius) so it can hold up better than most common beard oils. Shea butter is also considered a great heat protectant because its thermal conductivity is almost as good as popular silicones used in most heat protectants. There are actual products sold as "heat protectants" that you can apply specifically during your beard straightening process. Or, just use a beard oil/balm that has ingredients capable of standing up to high heat situations. (Shameless plug alert! All our beard oil blends use Argan oil as one of the three key carrier oils along with Jamaican Black Castor Oil which ALSO has a high smoke point, 392 degrees Fahrenheit. Our beard balms use those same oils plus shea butter. We feel setting your straightener to 375 will get the brush hot enough to do the job but not damage your hair while using ManBasics products. Here endeth the plug!)

The entire goal is to heat up your hair to make it pliable and then use a comb or brush to brush it straight.

The reason we like a high-quality beard straightening brush is because of the temperature control. If you are using a hair dryer you are manually attempting to control the temperature that hits your beard based on how long you blow the hot air in one spot. You are likely determining "hot enough" based on your pain tolerance for burning yourself. The difference between not hot enough to shape the beard and too hot to burn your skin and damage your beard could be seconds.

Not very precise.

A quality beard straightening brush should have temperature control settings allowing you to set the temperature to a number of different temps usually ranging from about 325 degrees Fahrenheit to 450 degrees Fahrenheit. We suggest starting at the lowest temperature setting and working your way up if needed, preferably not going over 375 and definitely not over 400.

There are basically two kinds of brush/combs out there – cheap ones and good ones, haha! The cheap ones will have a single flat heat plate with a slide on (generally plastic) attachment that is the comb/brush. So basically, you are passing a flat iron over your bear with a comb attached to keep the heating element off your face and to help straighten your beard.

These can work OK we guess, but a GOOD beard brush is not much more expensive and will a) do a better job and b) be safer for your beard.

A good beard straightening brush will have each individual tine with its own heating element. It will look like a large plastic tine and usually the heating element will look a different color.

Basically, it is plastic surrounding a ceramic tine. The plastic protects the heat from touching your face, as plastic is a poor conductor of heat, while the ceramic tine heats your hair, as the ceramic is a good conductor of heat. I'm sure you can see how this is a more precise and consistent way of getting the heat from the brush to your hair.

We also suggest getting a beard straightening brush that CAN get up to a higher temperature like 450 degrees Fahrenheit. You won't ever want to USE it at that temperature, but the higher heat capability likely means you have a stronger heating element. This is nice because as you brush through your beard you are diffusing heat from the brush to your beard. So, the brush is cooling slightly which means you will need to wait for it to heat back up as you make another pass. A cheap brush will turn your grooming into a arduous process. The stronger heating brush is a real time saver.

At <u>ManBasics</u> we have an extra "hack" when straightening our beard.   The tines on a beard straightener are very "course" or thick, because of the bulk in having the heating element in each tine.   So, while you are heating up your beard as you brush through it, you aren't particularly combing it very effectively.

We like to brush through our beard using the beard straightener with one hand and follow behind the beard straightening brush with our sandalwood comb.   This gives you the best of both worlds: a heated brush and a fine comb to affect the maximum number of beard hairs.

Make sure you are actually BRUSHING your beard . . . don't simply put the brush in one place and let it sit for a bit. You will almost certainly burn your beard. A little common sense goes a long way here, so just be careful brothers.

We think beard straighteners are pretty cool, but as we mentioned they can damage your beard. We don't recommend you using it every day.

Coloring Your Beard

Short answer? Don't do it.

Long answer? We think it is a bad idea and you shouldn't do it.

Firstly, your beard is a reflection of YOU . . . so why try and make it something it isn't? Is your beard grey? Guess what . . . it probably means you are getting old. Embrace it brother. Some might call it "mature", and women find maturity sexy.

Second, most beard coloring products are really harsh on you, your sking, and your beard. There's a reason that you where plastic gloves while using it and they don't want you having it make contact with your skin and they don't want you leaving it in too long . . . it's some harsh ass stuff brothers!

Plus, let's say you DO successfully manage to put it in without burning yourself.   Great, you've gone from looking 45 to 35 . . . for the week it takes for your beard to grow a little bit.   Now you've got grey roots and brown/black/whatever colored rest of your beard.   Now you either have to go and repeat the process again or look ridiculous (well, in our humble opinion).

Trust us guys.   That weird streak of grey doesn't look stupid. It looks awesome. The entire thing being white doesn't make you look old, it makes you look like freaking Gandalf man!   We'll support you in whatever beard you want guys, but please consider just letting your beard be itself. It will love you for it.

Beard Trimming Techniques – you may have noticed, we didn't really cover this topic . . . well, at all. I mean, we covered some of the beard styles and what they should look like, but not the specifics of trimming it to shape.

I wouldn't say that's really "by design" . . . but it did become a conscious decision as we got more and more into writing this tome.

Look, it's not 1975 where you buy a book and need step by step instructions with pictures. A picture is worth a thousand words, but VIDEO is worth millions. Trust us when we tell you that there are plenty of videos that can and will do a MUCH better job of instructing you on the best techniques to trim your beard.

Honestly, we just felt it would be a waste of both our times to attempt to tackle that subject. There are so many different ways to do it with a wide variety of particular tools (electric trimmers, scissors etc.) that it just makes sense to find the video instruction specific to the technique you are trying to find.

Beard Transplants

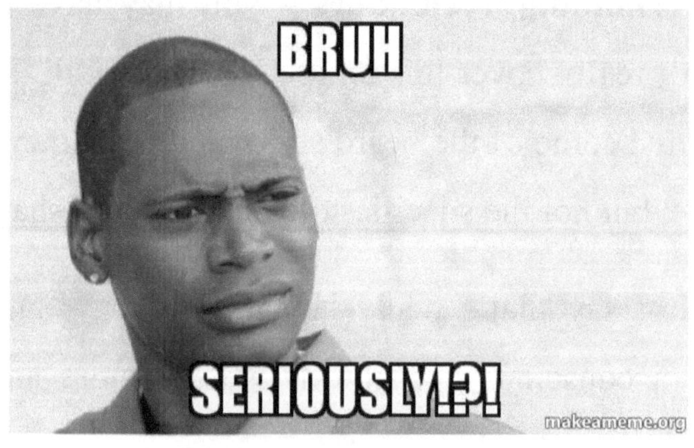

That's all we have to say about that.

Manly Salons

There's a relatively new phenomenon popping up around that you may have noticed: manly salons.

Basically, these are places you can go get your hair cut, but instead of sitting next to a mom bringing their three year old in for his first hair cut (who then starts screaming bloody murder as you sit there wishing the experience was over) you will sit next to other guys and they will offer you a beer while you wait. Sweet!

I told my wife about this place I had discovered and really built it up to the "And then they offered me a beer! Can you believe it!"

She stared at me blankly and said, "What do you think us girls do when we go get a manicure?" and then she walked off as I stood there stupid and speechless. Spoiler alert guys, your lady is WAY ahead of you. Mine is at least.

Anyway, these places tend not to just be a Sports Clips with booze. They really do cater to guys which means they have people on staff who can groom and maintain your beard if you so desire. They will likely have a true "barber" on staff who can do straight razor shaves as well (for those of you without full beards, or who like an edge up).

A wise man once said: Only do the things that only you can do. We heartily agree. If you can outsource a little beard maintenance and enjoy a social atmosphere and a cocktail all at once? Hell yes, we are on board. If you haven't found one of these yet in your home-town try googling "manly salon" and likely some place will come up like I'm describing. It's worth checking out.

Chapter Eleven - Go Forth and Grow

At <u>ManBasics</u> we think beards are like women: we love them in all shapes and sizes.

Mountain Man beard? You go Grizzly Adams.

Fu Man Chu? More like Fu Man WHOO!

Royale? We bow before your royal visage.

Goatee? Emphasis on G.O.A.T. Greatest of all time!

Pencil Thin Moustache? You are clearly aspiring to be a villain who chuckles evilly while twisting their 'stache. We love it.

Handlebar? We dig it hos.

Point is, whatever style you go for . . . do it well and let it be YOU.

Talk To Your Beard

OK, that may have come out wrong. LISTEN to your beard. There are lots of tips and tricks in this guide, but every person and every beard is different.

Your beard and face will let you know what it needs. Just be self-aware and we promise your beard will let you know what it needs. Hopefully this guide will serve as a translator to things your beard has already spoken up about.

Oh, and one last thing: Love your beard, it will love you back.

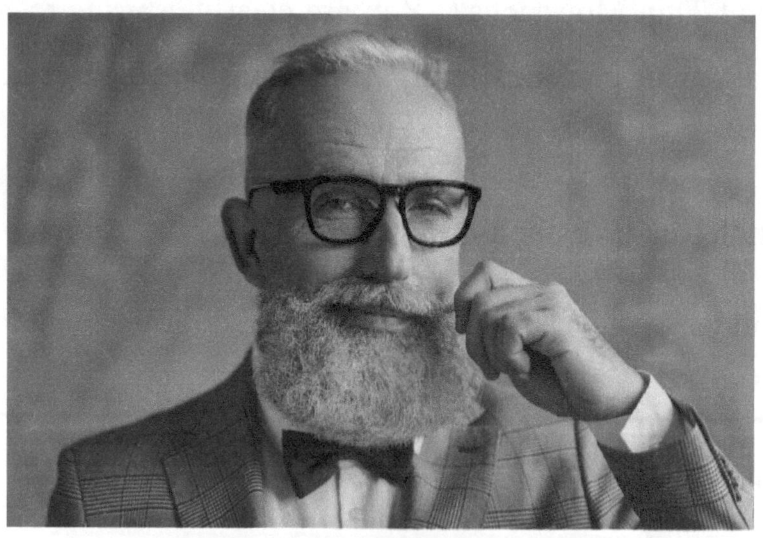

Figure 21 - Go forth and beard boldy brothers!

One Last Shameless Plug

Now that we have ended our tome, may we indulge in one last shameless plug? Nearly all of our knowledge and about beard care and maintenance has grown out of the experience of founding and running ManBasics, a men's personal care products company that specializes in sticking to the basics.

ManBasics produces men's personal care products that leave out the unnecessary elements and ingredients and sticks to the basics.

There are plenty of companies out there catering to men, there are plenty trying to be "all-natural" or "vegan" or "organic" . . . but our "just the basics" philosophy is built-in check that guides us. In some cases, it ALLOWS us to make a product that an "organic" company couldn't make. For example, our "naturally derived" deodorant. It's a spray deodorant, so it has water in it. Well, to be a responsible producer and create a product that is shelf-stable you have to have SOME sort of preservative in there, or you are gonna end up growing mold and making someone sick. In this case "the basics" INCLUDES putting in a preservative. We didn't waste time figuring out whether there SHOULD be a preservative, we spent that time researching what would be the BEST preservative for our clients. It's not all-natural or organic, but it IS the "basics" of what needs to be in there to keep it a viable product that people will want and can use. It is aluminum-free, paraben-free, alcohol-free, drug-free, sugar-free and drama free.

If all this sounds pretty cool to you, then please check us out on the web at:

www.ManBasics.com

Thanks, and beard on brothers!

Appendix – Great Beard Care Ingredients

There are a lot of great ingredients that can go into beard care products. Earlier we mentioned that we would compile some of these with their known benefits, so you have an idea what to look for in a beard oil or beard balm. The inclusion or exclusion of any of these ingredients does not in and of itself determine the worth of a product. That said, here are a few of our favorite ingredients.

Essential Oils

As discussed earlier, essential oils are the distilled "essence" of some sort of plant material. There is no doubt that natural materials affect our bodies in both positive and negative ways. Just try ingesting a raw, whole jalapeno and tell us your body wasn't affected in some way.

Yet, some are skeptics that natural materials can have similar *positive* effects as compared to the obvious negative ones.

We can sympathize with a degree of skepticism, but many modern day medicines are merely natural remedies with a dash of "science" added in.

For example, it has been relatively common knowledge for centuries that willow bark served as an effective pain reliever. Boiling willow bark tea was a common remedy for pain.

To make a long story short, willow bark extract was tweaked a bit to become what we know now as Aspirin.

We share this example to give a little perspective to those of you who may not have considered natural ingredients being capable of improving your life.

This will not be a complete list of essential oils and their benefits regarding your beard but is simply a few of our favorite ingredients that seem to be great for the health of your beard and face.

Rosemary Essential Oil – Rosemary is one of the best essential oils you can use for your beard, or any hair for that matter. Rosemary is said to:

- have anti-inflammatory properties
- promote nerve growth
- improve circulation

In a 2015 peer reviewed study Rosemary Essential Oil was found to be just as effective as Minoxidil in preventing hair loss, while another study showed that it actually promoted hair growth. It also side stepped a common issue with Minoxidil containing drugs (like Rogaine) . . . namely itchy scalp. So basically, with Rosemary you get the benefits of Minoxidil without negative side effects while staying all-natural and smelling nice. Sweet.

Peppermint Essential Oil - This essential oil is chock full of nutrients and minerals with fatty acids. Of course it also has that cooling effect from menthol, which you have probably experienced with some shampoo product in your life. Additionally, it also has antiseptic and antimicrobial properties, which help to cool the skin and sooth itchy skin or flaky beard.

Like Rosemary, Peppermint essential oil has ALSO proven to be as effective as Minoxidil in promoting hair growth and preventing hair loss . . . at least in mice.

A peer reviewed 2014 Korean study showed that peppermint essential oil showed more prominent hair growth in mice after 4 weeks than Minoxidil.

We think the menthol which gives that cool feeling actually stimulates the hair follicles, thereby promoting hair growth . . . but we aren't scientists (or mice for that matter). That said, we think Peppermint Essential Oil is Beard Growth Super Food.

Sandalwood Essential Oil – Sandalwood essential oil is a bit more complex. A recent German study showed that Sandalwood essential oil had REMARKABLE effects in growing hair by the multiplication of keratin in human skin cells.

That said, the study was a) using a synthetic version of sandalwood and b) conducted by the company producing said synthetic.

So, what LOOKS like promising research could be a bunch of self promoting horse crap.

That said, there is plenty of peer reviewed science that sandalwood prevents split ends in hair.   Also, Sandalwood is excellent for your skin. Sandalwood oil will soften and restore the skins ability to retain moisture. It is powerful for relieving rashes and inflammation and will also aid in scar fading, healing eczema, psoriasis, and soothing acne.

There is also a boatload of anecdotal evidence that Sandalwood smells f#$king awesome.

Oh, and one more thing: it's rumored to be an aphrodisiac. (we buried the lead).

Any Citrus Essential Oil – Orange, lime, lemon etc. are all citrus essential oils. They all have that . . . well, citrusy scent that we know and love and all share some common benefits to your skin and beard as well.

All citrus essential oils are astringent, which means it will tighten the skin slightly. This will help the skin look bright, toned and help eliminate wrinkles.

In addition, there's a reason almost every cleaning product you know has a version with a citrus scent: it's a natural antiseptic skin cleanser.

Carrier Oils

As we discussed there are plenty of great carrier oils out there. Using practically anything that is all natural and is helping to restore moisture to your face will be better than doing nothing, but we think certain carrier oils are the absolute best.

Jojoba Oil – This is an oil you have likely heard of before, at least in passing.   Jojoba oil is an all-natural oil that most closely mimics the "sebum" or oils our body produces naturally to keep our face moisturized.

So, while jojoba oil is a botanical substance, the chemical makeup is so similar to the oils your body naturally produces that your skin can't tell the difference. This makes it less likely to clog your pores, which is what leads to breakouts and less severe acne.

Jojoba oil is a "humectant" ingredient, meaning it helps to retain moisture, which if course is the entire point of using beard oil in the first place.

It is also full of vitamin E, which acts as a natural antioxidant. Vitamin E has long been used by health professionals to help with scarring. While this research is still ongoing, the results are promising that this is a real thing.

There is evidence that Jojoba oil also has anti-inflammatory properties that can help prevent psoriasis, eczema, and even acne.

Moroccan Argan Oil – Like Jojoba Oil, Argan oil is an abundant source of vitamin E as well as sporting a high content of antioxidants. In addition, it is full of oleic acid and linoleic acid. These oils have been shown to lubricate the hair shaft and help your hair maintain moisture (again, maintaining moisture is the whole reason we are using beard conditioner at all!)

The fatty acids in Argan oil are why Argan Oil has such a high smoke point. The fatty acids form a protective layer against heat, which makes it an ideal ingredient if you plan to use a beard straightener or any other heat application device to train your beard.

Jamaican Black Castor Oil - Black Castor Oil is created from the seeds of the castor bean which in the case of black castor oil are then roasted to extract the oil, which gives it the "black" namesake.

Black Castor Oil is a natural humectant, which like jojoba and Argan oils will promote hydration in your beard and face (what we want!).

Of course, it is LOADED with vitamins: Vitamin C, E, B6, B7 and uniquely includes a rich source of 90% Omega-9 fatty acids (ricinoleic) that helps to seal moisture into the hair.   This will help to thicken your beard while preventing damage and split ends.

Black Castor Oil is a relative "newbie" to the market (at least in terms of being well known), but there it a lot of anecdotal evidence about its efficacy in promoting hair growth. That's because it is rich in ricinoleic acid—a type of fatty acid found to fight inflammation.

When Black Castor Oil is applied it is purported to enhance the health of the hair follicles and, in turn, promote hair growth (as well as protect against hair loss).

Again, at this time the evidence is anecdotal, but we think the known benefits make this an ingredient well worth considering.

Also, Black Castor Oil is thicker than most other oils, which we think gives it a great "feel" when applying to our beard.

Coconut Oil – Also an excellent choice of carrier oil. Like so many oils, it is rich an vitamins like vitamin A, B, E, and K. Coconut oil also helps to prevent damage from the sun by forming a thin lipid layer. It also has a long shelf life, which makes it a popular choice amongst beard oil producers.

Almond Oil – Almond oil is quickly absorbed into the skin which makes it a great choice to quickly moisturize your beard and skin. It is also known for its ability to sooth inflamed skin, which makes it a great choice for beard growers with especially dry or irritated skin.

This list is by no means a comprehensive list, it's just a few of our favorites over at ManBasics.

Oh, did we mention that a good number of these ingredients can be found in our <u>all-natural beard oils and beard balms</u>? Feel free to check them out!